We dedicate this book to the great Danish strength
athlete Peter Jensen.

Improvised Isometric Exercise Devices™

The Daisy Chain

How a Simple Climber's Daisy Chain Can Become a Powerful Improvised Isometric Exercise Device or IIED™

Published by

MajorVision International

2020

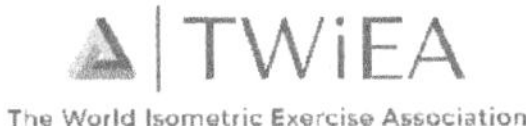

Approved by The World Isometric Exercise Association

www.HelenRenee.com – www.BrianSterlingVete.com

Contents

6. **Exercise Resources**
  - 1) Abdominals
    - Knee Raise and Trunk Curl
    - Trunk Curl Lying
    - The Side Bend
  - 2) Biceps
    - Biceps Curl Kneeling
    - Single Arm Kneeling Curl
    - Standing Leg-Resisted Curl
    - Standing Biceps Curl
    - Multi-Angle Standing Biceps Curl
  - 2 & 3) Biceps and Triceps Simultaneous
    - (Left and Right Side)
  - 3) Triceps
    - Forwards Triceps Press with Both Arms
    - Single Arm Forward Triceps Press
    - Overhead Triceps Press Single Arm
    - Triceps Forward Press Down Single Arm
    - Triceps Side Press Single Arm
  - 4) Back: Upper Chest-Level Pull-Apart
    - Chest-Level Upper-Back Pull-Apart
    - Overhead Upper-Back Pull-Apart
    - Seated Row
    - Standing Single Arm Row
  - 5) Lower Back:
    - Good Morning Overhead Pull-Apart
    - The Deadlift

- 6) Chest:
  - Chest Cross-Press
  - Across Back Flye
  - Standing Chest Press
  - Resisted Push-up
- 7) Shoulders:
  - Side Lateral Raise
  - Side Lateral Raise Cross Foot Loops
  - Front Raise
  - Single-Arm Standing Press
  - Carabiner Linking
  - Climber's Sling Looping
  - Upright Row
- 8) Thighs Front:
  - Wall Squat and Leg Press
  - The Squat
  - Forward Split Squat
  - Leg Extension
  - The Abductor
- 8 & 9) Thighs Simultaneous Front and Rear:
  - Leg Extension and Leg Curl Combined
- 9) Thigh Hamstring:
  - Leg Curl Against Wall
- 10) Calf:
  - Immovable Object Heel Raise-Push

7. Conclusion

- What is TWiEA™?

Important General Safety and Health Guidelines

This disclaimer applies to all content contained within or associated with this book, including but not limited to: books, courses, articles, publications of any kind, videos, associated websites, recommendations, suggestions, coaching, and any advice whether written, digital, verbal, or otherwise, created or delivered by Brian Sterling-Vete and Helen Renée Wuorio, who are the copyright holders, creators, instructors, and originators of the material herein.

Medical Approval Required

You must not undertake any exercise programme, course, or dietary change referenced in this book or related materials without first obtaining full approval from a qualified medical doctor. Only your doctor is able to determine your suitability for the physical activities or dietary practices described, particularly if you have any known or suspected medical conditions, are pregnant, or have other significant health concerns.

You are strongly advised to present all relevant content from this book, including any associated videos, audio material, or online content, to your doctor for review and to obtain their written or verbal approval prior to beginning any exercise or diet plan.

Not a Substitute for Personalised Professional Advice

The exercises, plans, recommendations, and suggestions provided are intended solely as general reference material. They are not tailored to individual circumstances and do not constitute professional, personalised medical or fitness advice. They must not be relied upon as a replacement for a qualified personal trainer, fitness coach, dietitian, or medical professional. This material is not intended for use by children, and all exercise equipment should be kept out of reach of minors.

Exercise Caution and Equipment Safety

You must always exercise caution and avoid overexertion. If you experience any pain, discomfort, shortness of breath, chest pain, irregular heartbeat, faintness, dizziness, nausea, or any other concerning symptom, stop exercising immediately and seek medical assistance without delay.

Before each use, you must thoroughly inspect all exercise equipment—whether purpose-made or improvised—as well as any doorways, frames, floors, benches, chairs, or furniture used for exercising. Equipment should only be used if it is in proper working order, free from visible damage or wear, and securely positioned to avoid injury.

Always take care when transitioning into or out of exercise positions, particularly when moving to and from the floor or using any surfaces or objects for support.

Limitation of Liability

Neither Brian Sterling-Vete nor Helen Renée Wuorio, nor any person, company, or organisation associated with them, accepts any liability for injury, loss, harm, illness, damage to property, or any other adverse outcome—whether direct or indirect—arising from the use of any information, recommendations, exercises, or materials contained in this book or any related content, including websites and videos.

Further Guidance

For further general health and fitness information, we recommend consulting reputable sources such as:

The National Health Service (UK): https://www.nhs.uk/Livewell/fitness/pages/physical-activity-guidelines-for-adults.aspx

The Mayo Clinic (USA): https://www.mayoclinic.org/healthy-lifestyle

Chapter 1: Isometrics and IIEDs

This series of books is about what we call IIEDs, or Improvised Isometric Exercise Devices. These books are not intended to be workout routines. Instead, they are a resource demonstrating several valid exercise ideas that can be performed with a specific IIED. Also, since one of the great benefits of isometric exercises is that they can be performed almost anywhere, we will demonstrate the exercises in common surroundings.

One of the wonderful things about isometric exercise is that it can be performed effectively without using any cumbersome gym equipment or anything else for that matter. I am certain that hundreds of thousands, perhaps even several million people, perform daily isometric exercise routines using only their arms, legs and body as the counterbalancing immovable object required to perform an isometric exercise contraction during a self-resisted workout session.

I am one of those people who frequently perform self-resisted isometric exercises. Therefore, I also know precisely how deceptively powerful self-resistance or any other type of isometric exercise can be. This is because once you have set your muscles into a biomechanically correct position to perform an exercise, the results obtained from that exercise are directly proportionate to the effort, applied force, and overall level of intensity. The more you input, the greater the resulting output; it is that simple.

Therefore, the same isometric exercises can be performed with equal effectiveness by a completely unfit beginner who is middle-aged or a young professional athlete who is at the peak of their performance potential. It is all about who applies the most effort, force, and intensity.

Theoretically, the beginner, in my analogy, could even derive far more benefit from the same exercises than the professional athlete. This would be if the beginner applied their maximum safe level of effort, force, and intensity to the same exercises that the professional athlete did not take seriously and performed only a fraction of their potential force and overall intensity. It is a universal constant that no matter what exercise system you perform or what equipment you choose to use, the results you get are always going to be directly proportionate to the effort, force, and overall intensity that is applied.

Even though isometric exercises can be effectively performed in a self-resisted way without any equipment, sometimes, using equipment might be beneficial and interesting. Even using some basic improvised exercise equipment can allow you to apply greater force and intensity to certain exercises and perform a wider variety of exercises.

Today, there is a greater choice of proprietary isometric and isotonic/isometric exercise equipment than ever before. Also, most, if not all, of these devices are excellent, well-made, durable, and functional. We would include devices such as the Iso-Bow®, the Bullworker®, the Steel Bow® and the Iso-Gym® in this category, and we will give you a comprehensive overview of each of these devices in a later section. However, in this book, we are going to focus on the simple climber's daisy chain and how it can be used as a highly effective and extremely versatile IIED.

Daisy Chains as IIEDS

A Typical Climber's Daisy Chain

Note the Foot Loop at One End and the Carabiner Point/s at the Other End

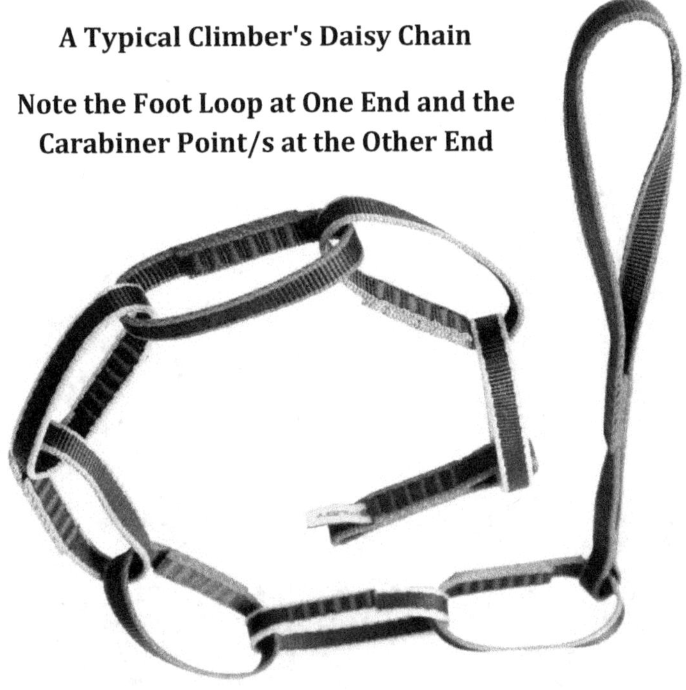

For those who do not know, a daisy chain is an item of basic climbing equipment. It is a webbing strap that is several feet/centimetres long. Typically, it is made from approximately one-inch (2.54 cm) nylon webbing of the same or similar type to that used in climbing slings and lengthening straps between anchor points and the main climbing rope. The webbing is securely stitched at intervals of approximately two inches to form loops on one side along the length of the main webbing strap.

Alternatively, and these are the type we prefer, the nylon webbing is sewn into a series of closely spaced interlocked loops to create a looped daisy chain for the

16

desired length of the device. At one end, there is usually a much larger foot loop to accommodate a climbing boot, and at the other end, there is a carabiner point made from a smaller piece of nylon webbing in a tight loop or bite. These are either the same as or closely resemble a climber's device known as a screamer.

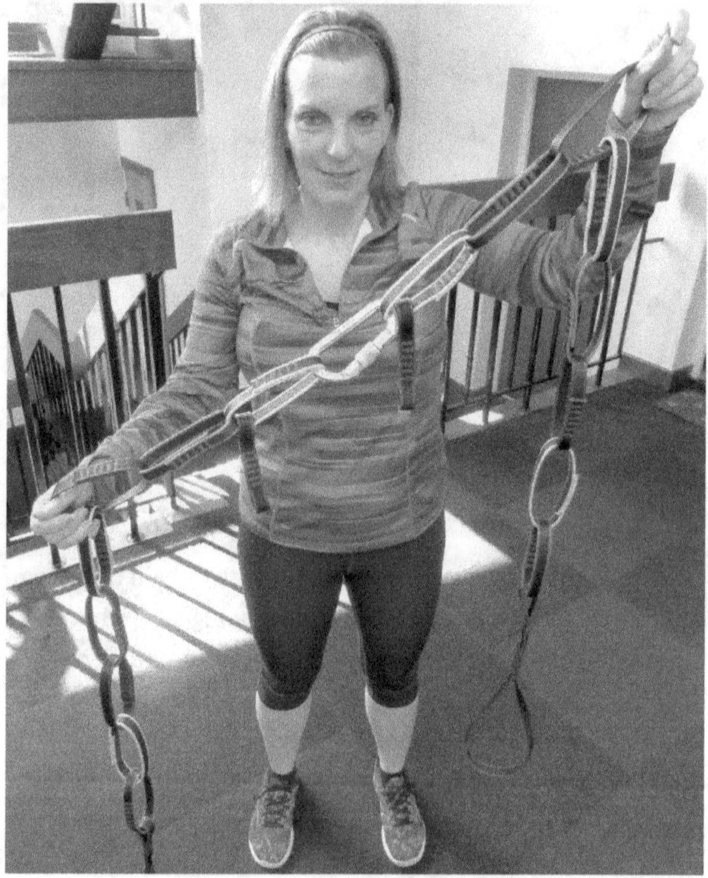

Two Daisy Chains Linked Together by Carabiner

From a climbing perspective, the closely spaced loops allow a climber to fine-tune the length from the sit-harness to the anchor, thereby allowing the best possible reach for the next placement. Daisy chains are particularly useful because they can be easily extended by clipping one to another using a carabiner. Also, a climbing sling can be interlocked securely through any of the daisy chain loops.

Daisy chains are extremely strong, with a typical average breaking strength of at least 22 kilonewtons or 4,900 lbf. To give you an idea of the strength of a daisy chain, 22 Kilonewtons (kN) equals 2,243 Kilograms of Force (kgf) or 4944.96 lbs, with 1 kN = 101.97 kgf and 1 kgf = 0.009807 kN. To give you a better frame of reference for the breaking strain of a 22 kN daisy chain, an average Range Rover Sport SUV weighs about 4,727 lb or 2,144 kg. Therefore, a typical 22 kN daisy chain made from nylon webbing can be used safely as an IIED or any other kind of exercise, for that matter. When undamaged and properly made, they cannot be ripped apart during exercise or anything else, even by The World's Strongest Man.

A key feature of the daisy chain is its ability to be used in a multitude of exercises, much like a barbell or a dumbbell. The closely spaced daisy chain loops make excellent handgrips along the entire length of the daisy chain, providing you with a comfortable and effective workout tool. This versatility is what sets them apart and makes them a valuable asset in any fitness arsenal.

The benefits of using daisy chains in specific exercises are numerous. The ready-made foot loop at one end of the device allows for a wide variety of isometric exercises to be performed while standing upright or seated on the floor or bench. Using the foot anchor technique, many traditional-style exercises can then be performed.

These include the squat, the split squat, the deadlift, the good morning, the side lateral raise, the front raise, the single-arm curl, the double-arm curl, the upright rowing and shrugs, etc. This practical application of daisy chains in various exercises is what makes them a versatile and effective tool in any workout routine.

When looped around the back and shoulders, certain exercises can be performed, including the triceps press-down, the triceps front-press, and the triceps side-press. Also, when wrapped around the width of the back and shoulders, exercises like the chest press, chest flyes, and single-arm triceps press. Also, when lying face-down on the floor with a daisy chain across the back, then a resisted isometric push-up chest press can be performed at various positions on the ROM or Range of Motion.

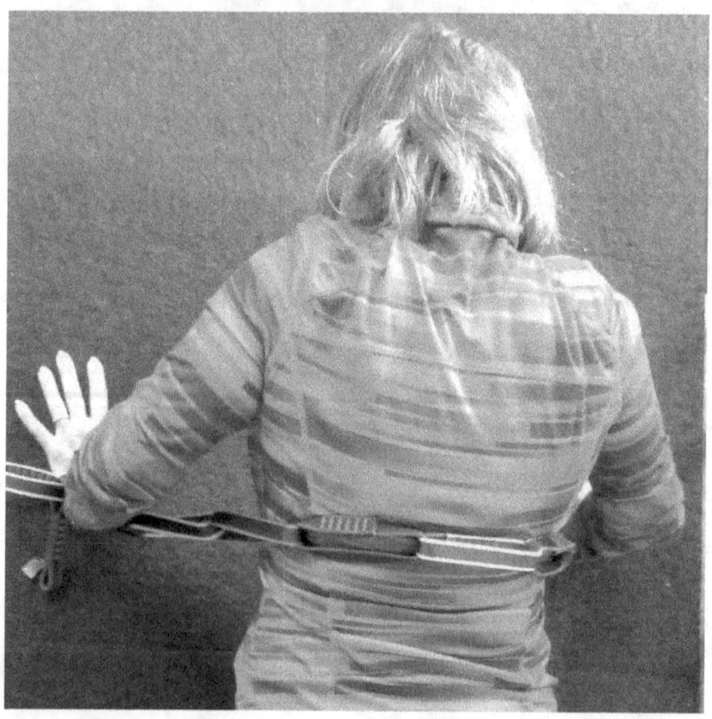

There are more advanced options for those who possess at least a reasonable knowledge of exercise performance science and biomechanics. These are when a daisy chain is used to create legitimate exercise positions that are biomechanically correct, while, at the same time, they are also extremely biomechanically disadvantageous from an exercise performance perspective. For example, you can easily achieve an acute elbow angle to perform a triceps forward press, extension, or pushdown.

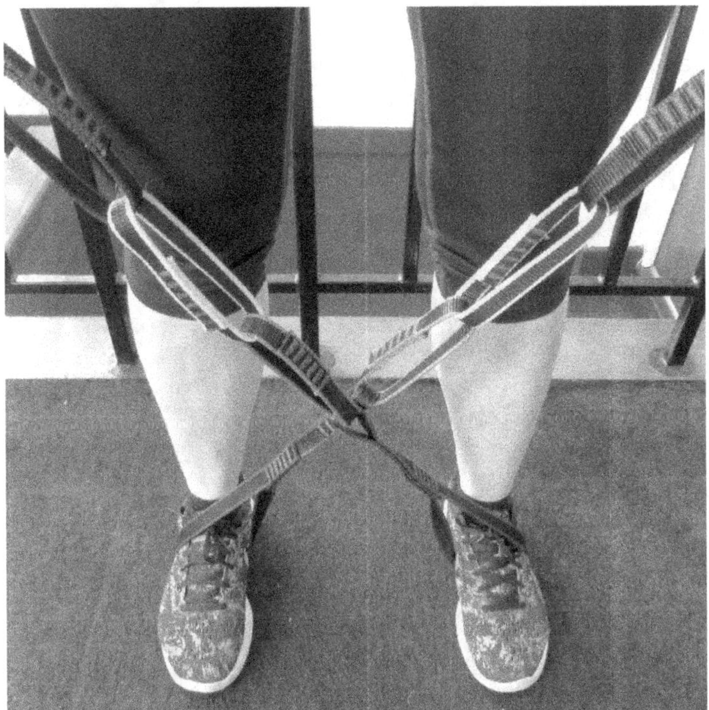

Adding a simple daisy chain to your exercise equipment arsenal opens up a world of possibilities. Suddenly, you have a multitude of additional exercise options and variations at your disposal. These are only limited by the number of variations that can be imagined by combining a good knowledge of correct exercise biomechanics and muscle actions with how various parts of the body or other fixed objects can secure the daisy chain. This versatility is what makes daisy chains a game-changer in your workout routine.

Therefore, in the exercise section of this book, we will provide a comprehensive resource list. These show how to perform a wide range of exercises for each of the main body parts/muscle groups with a daisy chain or pair of daisy chains. Where appropriate, we will also show exercise variations with additional climbing slings either looped together or secured by a carabiner to form different lengths added to the daisy chain.

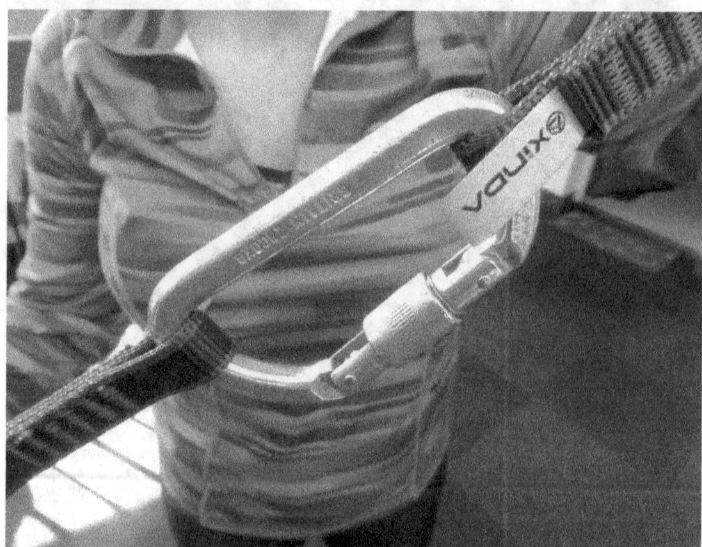

Since a comprehensive total-body workout can be performed in as few as 10 exercises, you can choose a single exercise from each section to devise your ideal total-body exercise routine. Alternatively, if desired, more than one exercise can be performed from each section to expand the

21

workout to exercise a wider range of muscles from different angles/positions.

For advanced users, each exercise can also be performed at more than one point on the limb's ROM, or Range of Motion. This will develop a more even strength curve on the limb's ROM, which many advanced athletes and sports enthusiasts/professionals will find extremely useful. In short, your options are extremely varied and highly effective; the choice of what you use is yours.

For those who do not already know, before we get to the exercise section, we will explain a little more about the science behind it all, the background of the system, etc. This section about isometric exercise science is similar to those in our other books.

This is because isometric exercise science is always going to be the same. The only variables between books are the exercises being performed and the isometric exercise devices used.

This is a condensed section in comparison to books such as The Isometric Bible™, which goes into much more detail about different isometric techniques, and The 70 Second Difference™, which has a comprehensive section on exercise and even bigger sections on advanced nutrition.

Chapter 2: Exercise Science Overview

In this chapter, we will provide a user-friendly overview of exercise science and discuss the features and benefits of various exercise techniques and concepts. For those who want more in-depth information about the science of isometric exercise and health and fitness in general, we suggest that you also read our books The ISOmetric Bible™ and The 70 Second Difference™. Both are available on Amazon.

Walking as Exercise

Walking is a vastly underrated form of exercise; even a short, regular daily walk can yield tremendous health benefits. In recent years, several notable studies have been performed on the health-related benefits of walking and how walking can even help prevent many serious diseases and illnesses.

In the journal Healthy Heart for Life!, Dr Martha Grogan of the Mayo Clinic in Rochester, Minnesota, said that research indicates that walking for just 10 minutes a day can halve one's risk of having a heart attack. She also noted that a sedentary lifestyle increases the risk of a heart attack almost as much as smoking does.

Therefore, given that golf typically involves walking far longer than just 10 minutes a day, even golfers are dramatically cutting their risk of a heart attack while simultaneously having fun. Whereas Nordic Walkers and Trekkers naturally gain even greater health-related benefits due to the greater distances they walk.

In Great Britain, the NHS research indicates the same as the Mayo Clinic research. After the results of an extensive international study were published, the National Health Service highly recommends walking as an excellent form of exercise that helps to prevent several serious illnesses and diseases.

Other studies focused on adults with a high risk of type 2 diabetes and heart disease. Research has found that an additional 2,000 steps per day lowered the risk of experiencing a cardiac issue by up to 10% for this group of people. Furthermore, continuing research indicated that for every additional 2,000 steps per day that were taken, the risk was further reduced by 8%. The research was carried out by teams from the NIHR Leicester-Loughborough Diet, Lifestyle, and Physical Activity Biomedical Research Unit, the University of Leicester, and Duke University School of Medicine in the USA. They also collaborated with other researchers from universities and institutes around the world. The results were published in the medical journal The Lancet.

Research indicates that two and a half hours of walking each week can also help to reduce the risk of contracting seven types of cancer. The research suggested that it reduced the risk of kidney cancer in both sexes by 11 per cent and by 17 per cent if the length of time spent walking/taking moderate exercise was increased to five hours per week. The research also suggested that two and a half hours of walking each week could reduce the risk of contracting breast cancer by 5%, and by 10% for five hours of walking per week. Women were up to 18% less likely to get cancer of the womb, both sexes were less likely to get non-Hodgkin's lymphoma, up to 19 per cent less likely to contract myeloma, and men were up to 14% less likely to get colon cancer. The details of the study were published in the Journal of Clinical Oncology.

Walking Vs Running as a Fat Burner

Walking and running are both excellent ways to get fitter, burn calories, tone up, and promote weight loss. There are different and distinct benefits to each, which we will briefly touch on. Running burns more calories than walking does. However, walking burns more fat than running does. So, it is a trade-off, especially since walking more will increase your N.E.A.T. factor. We will explain more about N.E.A.T. in the next section.

When exercising at a lower intensity, fat is used as the body's primary fuel. When you shift gears and increase the pace from walking to running, your body burns more carbohydrates as fuel.

However, it does not matter too much whether you are burning body fat or carbohydrates as the primary fuel. What is important is that you burn the most calories possible during your exercise session and stimulate a long-term increase in your Base Metabolic Rate. Therefore, even though walking may burn more stored fat as fuel, running will still burn more overall calories.

Another important factor to consider when comparing the differences between walking and running is the risk of injury. Running carries more risk of injury than walking, so the choice is yours.

Walking, General Activity and N.E.A.T. - Non-Exercise Activity Thermogenesis

The acronym N.E.A.T. is becoming increasingly discussed in relation to weight control, body fat, and exercise. The N.E.A.T. acronym stands for Non-Exercise Activity Thermogenesis, and it comes from Dr James Levine's research into how we expend calories.   In simple terms, it means: "burning calories through daily life, and not through exercise," and in the simplest terms, it means that people who are active and move around a lot burn more calories and tend to be slimmer than people who do not.

There are two basic ways in which we burn calories. One is while we exercise, and the other is through the general activities of daily living. The key question is: "Which, if any, is more important to weight loss, and what are the levels of body fat that we carry?" According to Dr Levine, it is the N.E.A.T. that appears to be far more important for calorie burning than dedicated exercise time. Dr Levine's research also led to the phrase "Being Active Naturally" becoming more commonly used.

Providing that you exercise good judgment in your food choices and the macros around proper portion control, in addition to your regular exercise routine, just being a little more active in everyday life will make a huge difference in terms of weight control and overall body fat levels.

In our opinion, N.E.A.T. alone is not a great panacea when it comes to losing weight and staying slim. After all, when people are stressed and mentally fatigued because of a tough workday, it is not always easy to opt for the most sensible food choices, nor is it likely that you will want to go out and do something active to increase your daily movement factor. However, N.E.A.T. is certainly something to be factored into your overall lifestyle because it makes a significant difference to your overall appearance and fitness levels.

The Basic Types of Resistance Exercise

All muscle training falls into two or three specific categories, depending on how you break them down. In the most basic form, there are two types: contraction with or without movement. Breaking them down a step further, there become three categories, with one being isotonic, another isokinetic, and last but certainly not least, isometric.

Isotonic training is all about movement, with muscle shortening and lengthening during the lifting and lowering phases of the exercise. We know that the isotonic category can be broken down further into three parts. One part is the concentric contraction, which is the lifting phase of an exercise when the muscles shorten. Another is the eccentric phase, the lowering part of an exercise when the muscles lengthen.

Lastly, the isotonic category includes the isokinetic contraction. In this contraction, the muscle changes in length during both the concentric and eccentric phases; however, the velocity remains constant no matter how much force is applied during the exercises.

Then comes the isometric category. With an isometric exercise, there is no movement whatsoever. To help you envision this, I will take a random weight training or freehand callisthenic exercise, such as a chest press, because it can be performed either with movement OR without movement as an isometric exercise.

For example, a barbell, a machine, or your bodyweight can be lifted and lowered to perform an exercise such as a barbell curl. This is called isotonic exercise, callisthenics, or simply exercise with movement.

To perform the same or similar exercise isometrically, you would attempt to perform the same or similar biomechanically correct actions of a barbell curl. However, at a certain point, or points if multiple exercise points were being used, the curling movement would stop because an immovable object point had been reached.

At that point or points, you would apply an increasing level of force until you reach the desired target level as you attempt to perform the curling exercise against the immovable object.

At the desired isometric exercise point, a constant force is applied against the immovable object for 7 seconds, which is the optimum isometric exercise time. The ideal basic isometric exercise point for general exercise is roughly at the mid-point when your muscles reach a stalemate working against each other or an immovable object. This is called a Standard isometric Contraction.

The harder you engage your muscles as you try to break the stalemate by lifting, pushing, or pulling, the stronger your muscles become. In doing so, you engage many more muscle fibres than normal as you attempt to move the immovable object and perform the curling exercise action.

Doors, desks, chairs, walls, and many other everyday items can serve as immovable objects. However, the simplest and most accessible immovable object is often yourself, making isometric exercise a convenient and empowering choice.

Isometric Overview

As you now know, isometric exercise does not involve any movement. Instead, the joint angle and the muscle length do not change during contraction. You also now know that 7 seconds is regarded as the optimum time to perform an isometric exercise.

However, almost everyone tends to count the exercise elapsed time much faster than the real elapsed time when exercising. This means that it is easy not to reach the magic 7 seconds of the optimum isometric exercise time. Therefore, we always suggest aiming to perform the exercise for 10 seconds to ensure that the 7-second target is always reached, even when under the stress of intense exercise.

Isometric exercise has been extensively scientifically researched and repeatedly proven to be a highly effective method for building strength and muscle. It is one of the most thoroughly researched exercise systems despite being one of the most misunderstood. This is likely due to fear, professional ignorance, and financial reasons, but the evidence of its effectiveness is undeniable.

The isometric exercise system can use several different techniques. Most of these techniques are highly advanced and intended for competitive athletes, martial arts practitioners, strength athletes, and bodybuilders. Therefore, they are not appropriate for a general isometric exercise session for the average person who simply wants to get stronger and fitter.

However, purely out of interest, I will list them here in case any fitness enthusiasts, athletes, or bodybuilders read this book and wish to try them. They are described in greater detail in our book called The Isometric Bible, which is available on Amazon and in good bookstores. The most common and advanced isometric exercise techniques include the following:

- Standard Isometric Contraction
- Yielding Isometric Contraction
- Maximum Duration Isometrics
- Oscillatory Isometrics
- Impact Absorption Isometrics
- Explosive Isometrics, AKA: Ballistic Isometrics
- Static-Dynamic Isometric
- Contrast Isometric
- Functional Isometrics
- TRISOmetrics™

More than enough isometric exercises can be performed without any equipment to allow a total body workout routine to be completed relatively easily. These will typically be self-resisting isometric exercises, which are excellent. However, by using only minimal readily available equipment such as walking poles, golf clubs, martial arts belts, climbing ropes, scuba diving webbing, weight belts, and broom handles, etc., it is possible to greatly expand the number of exercises that can be performed.

It is also perfectly possible to adapt and use other readily available items such as tow ropes, steel chains, towels, and commonly found immobile objects such as sturdy fixed barrier railings, solid walls, solid doors, door frames, or parked vehicles to perform a complete isometric exercise routine. Again, these are all excellent improvised exercise tools that allow an expanded range of highly effective isometric exercises to be performed.

Using improvised exercise tools can yield an unexpected additional benefit. This is because it allows one to focus more and apply greater concentration to each exercise. This is particularly useful for those who are either completely new to or are relatively new to the isometric exercise system. We will explain more about what these can be later in the book.

One of the things we love about both the isometric and self-resisted exercise systems is that as you get stronger through exercise, you can apply more force and intensity to your isometric or self-resisted exercises.

This, in turn, means that you can gradually increase the level of force and intensity you can safely apply to each exercise, which will mean that the results and benefits you receive will grow in a compound way through regular daily use. This is what we call a natural Adaptive Response™ mechanism, which is a useful aspect of our biology.

Isometric Exercise Science

Even until the mid-20th century, almost no scientific research had been performed on the benefits of isometric exercise. We also know that before the first serious scientific research study, people were trained isometrically by performing what we now call endurance isometrics.

Thankfully, isometric exercise has been thoroughly scientifically researched and proven for several decades. I would estimate that at least as much scientific research has been performed on it as on traditional resistance training.

The first major in-depth study into isometric exercise was performed at the world-famous Max Planck Institute in Dortmund, Germany. If you already have a reasonable knowledge of science, you will also know that the Max Planck Institute is a world-renowned centre of scientific excellence in many disciplines.

Between 1953 and 1958, one of the most extensive research studies was commissioned into isometric exercise science. Many consider these experiments to be the original gold standard of isometric exercise studies. The results were made widespread public knowledge in the resultant ground-breaking book, The Physiology of Strength, by Dr Theodor Hettinger, Research Fellow at the Max Planck Institute. During that 5-year research period, Dr Hettinger and Dr Muller performed a widely reported, reputed 5,500 experiments, although this figure is almost certainly apocryphal because they would have had to perform a minimum of three experiments a day, every day for five years.

Research suggests that the actual number of experiments performed by Hettinger and Muller was probably less than 50. However, many thousands of studies have almost certainly been completed at other institutions worldwide since then. These were conducted on male and female volunteers from all walks of life and at every level of strength, fitness, and athletic ability. Perhaps what surprised people the most was how dramatic and impressive the results were gained from performing isometric exercises. Also, because the same or similar results were easily repeatable, the data gained from the experiments was exceptionally reliable. The conclusion of the extensive studies proved beyond doubt the overall superiority of isometric exercise in building strength and muscle compared to traditional isotonic exercise methods. It also proved that the isometric system delivered these results much faster and with far less exercise than traditional resistance training.

Another extremely interesting result emerged from the experiments. This was because the optimum results were not produced by the length of time an isometric exercise was held, but by the correct level of force applied for a specific optimum time.

They found that performing only one daily isometric exercise for between 6 and 7 seconds and at only two-thirds of an individual's maximum effort could increase strength by an average of up to 5% per week. By any standards, strength gains of 5% in exchange for the expenditure of only 66%, or around two-thirds of an individual's maximum capacity, is an excellent result.

Perhaps even more amazingly, they discovered that after someone has performed a single 7-second training stimulus (exercise) per day, the muscle being exercised in that same position was no longer responsive to further gains. In other words, it did not matter how many more times you exercised the same muscle in the same position; there would be no further increase in muscle growth or strength. The only way to do this was to perform another isometric exercise at a different position, only the limb's ROM (Range Of Motion). The scientific data about this can be referenced on pages 28 to 31 of Dr Theodor Hettinger's book, "The Physiology of Strength."

In 2001, Nicolas Babault, PhD of the University of Burgundy, Dijon, France, led a team of scientists to research and examine how many muscle fibres were activated and how long they remained active during both traditional weight training and isometric training.

(The scientific research paper is published: Nicolas Babault, Michel Pousson, Yves Ballay, and Jacques Van Hoecke - Groupe Analyse du Mouvement, Unite´ de Formation et de Recherche Sciences et Techniques des Activite´s Physiques et Sportives, Universite´ de Bourgogne, BP 27877, 21078 Dijon Cedex, France.)

They discovered that when training intensely and in near-perfect style, the levels of muscle activation during repetitions of optimum maximal weight training were between 89.7% during the concentric contraction, or when lifting a weight, and 88.3% during the eccentric contraction, or when lowering a weight. For practical purposes, an average of about 89% overall.

The study also revealed that during the lifting, or concentric part of the exercise, the maximum intramuscular tension only lasted for between 0.25 and 0.5 seconds. For practical purposes, this is an average of about 1/3rd of a second during each isotonic repetition. This is because traditional isotonic resistance exercises naturally involve movement. They also have aspects of velocity and acceleration to consider in the overall equation. "Force" is only produced for a split second to produce a maximal contraction of the muscle fibres. The same research also showed that the level of muscle activation during isometric exercise was as high as 95.2% and that it lasted for the entire 7 to 10 seconds of each exercise. This is a huge increase over the 1/3rd of a second muscular activation achieved during a single repetition of weight training.

Therefore, based on these discoveries, technically, a single isometric exercise performed at only two-thirds of an individual's maximum can deliver similar or often even better results than the equivalent of up to 3 sets of 10 weight training repetitions in the lifting phase of the exercise.

To explain this further, I will use a typical barbell curl exercise in the lifting phase as my example, where the object of the exercise is to engage as many muscle fibres as possible in a maximum muscular contraction. Naturally, 3 sets of 10 repetitions give us an overall total of 30 repetitions. One set of 10 repetitions of the barbell curl in perfect high-intensity style produces a maximum muscular engagement for approximately 3.3 seconds. Three sets of 10 repetitions of the same exercise, a total of 30 repetitions, will give a total of approximately 9.9 seconds of maximum muscular engagement and an average of 89% muscle activation overall.

In comparison, one high-intensity isometric contraction exercise produces a maximum muscular engagement that lasts for the entire duration of the exercise. Even though the optimum time over which an isometric exercise is performed was found to be 7 seconds, this is almost always rounded up to the 10-second target number. The maximum muscular engagement will last for the entire 10 seconds of a high-intensity isometric exercise, with 95.2% muscle activation overall.

This is proof that is based entirely on scientific research that 3 sets of 10 near-perfect high-intensity curls when weight training, which takes several minutes to perform, still was not quite equal to the results achieved by a single 10-second high-intensity isometric curl exercise.

The Standard Isometric Contraction

The standard isometric contraction is a simple and highly effective technique. Therefore, we will focus on it for practical isometric training.

The standard isometric contraction, AKA: overcoming isometric contraction, AKA: maximum-effort isometrics, or whatever else you wish to call it, is when a muscle is applying force to push or pull against an immovable resistance. This is the most basic of all kinds of isometric exercise, and it is highly effective. This type of isometric contraction exercise was performed during the experiments by Dr T. Hettinger and Dr E. Muller at the Max

Planck Institute. It is also the technique referred to in their book The Physiology of Strength.

In a standard isometric contraction, it is theoretically possible to exert up to 100% of one's maximum capacity effort against an immovable object and then continue to hold that level of force throughout the exercise. This means that standard isometric contraction can be a very high-intensity exercise system.

Performing an isometric exercise against an immovable object at a certain level of force for a given duration of time will teach your body to recruit more muscle fibres to try to move the object. As you perform the exercise and generate as much force as possible, your CNS, or Central Nervous System, learns that it needs to activate and recruit more muscle fibres to reach the goal of moving the object.

Since this will naturally be impossible to move, the process will continue each time you exercise to make you stronger and grow more muscle. Your body mechanisms become trained to readily activate and recruit additional muscle fibres when facing similar challenges, which, in turn, repeats the cycle more readily every time.

As we mentioned earlier, the immovable/solid object can be anything completely solid and safe to use. This can be a wall, a door, a door jamb, a parked motor vehicle or anything similar. Perhaps the most common objects used to enhance everyday isometric exercise training are sturdy towels, climbing ropes, martial arts belts, scuba diving weight belts, webbing straps, golf clubs, and broom handles, etc. All the aforementioned items are excellent when used properly and will deliver some excellent results. More importantly, they are typically readily available for most people, which makes exercising with them so much easier.

Another common way to perform isometric exercise is to do it in a self-resisted way. Self-resisting means pushing or pulling against your limbs/hands/feet, etc. For example, you might place the palms of your hands together at chest level with your hands roughly at the midpoint of your body. In that position, you would then press your hands together using your chest muscles to provide the primary driving force, and then you would perform a highly effective self-resisted isometric chest press!

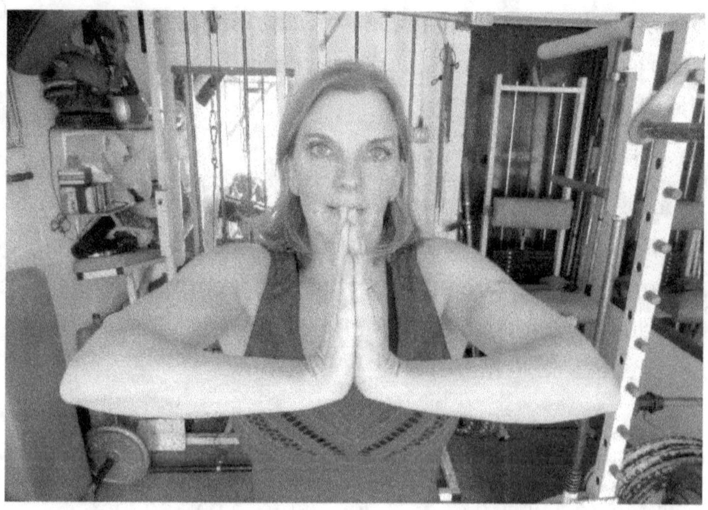

It is possible to perform a well-balanced and highly effective self-resisted isometric workout to exercise virtually every section of the body. So, never underestimate self-resistance exercise because it can be immensely powerful indeed. Also, self-resistance exercises are an excellent way

39

to ensure that a personal maximum resistance is used safely and with minimum risk of injury caused by applying too much force.

The fact is that it does not matter which method is chosen. It can be isometrics performed against an immovable object, self-resisted isometrics, or a combination of the two. The most important thing is that either the object must be completely immovable through human muscle power alone, or the force of one body part must be able to completely counterbalance the force of another body part to produce a muscular stalemate.

Intensity, Force, Strength, and Power

Intensity will always be a relative term, and it is often completely misunderstood when used regarding exercise. When it comes to exercising your muscles, intensity is the percentage of your ability to move a resistance. Technically, an individual's highest possible level of intensity is when they reach a point of momentary failure after exerting themselves completely.

However, the important questions we need to try to answer are: "How hard is hard?" and "How intense is intense?" To some degree, both are very subjective. Taking two people of roughly equal fitness, something that is intense to one person might be considered comparatively easy to the other.

Hard is a relative term, and handling 50 lbs of resistance is impossibly hard if your strength is only at the level required to lift 49 lbs. However, if you can lift 100 lbs as a maximum, then lifting 50 lbs is going to be comparatively easy.

Often, the only factors differentiating between people and the intensity level exerted are mental toughness, determination, and perception.

Therefore, to gain the greatest benefits from isometric exercise, the first thing that must be learned is how to determine, with a reasonable degree of accuracy, what level of intensity is being applied to an exercise.

It is just a fact that what one person deems to be 100% of their capacity will always be quite different from another person's estimate. The accurate estimation of what one person deems to be 2/3rds of their overall maximum intensity will also vary from person to person. The accuracy of estimation will also vary greatly between an experienced professional athlete and an absolute beginner to exercise.

Experience has taught us that most people who are new to exercise will always fall well short of accurately estimating any given percentage. A beginner will find it more challenging to accurately estimate what 2/3rds of their 100% maximum is compared to a more experienced athlete. Many people might believe they are performing at 100% capacity when they are only performing at around 2/3rds, or perhaps at only 50% or less of their 100% maximum.

This is because exercise is new to them, and therefore, the experiences and feelings in their bodies associated with it are also new. They simply have no common frame of reference when it comes to calculating/estimating their level of physical exertion.

The human brain has a built-in mechanism that helps to protect the body and prevent it from performing a physical activity to such a level that it could cause serious damage or even death. This is the mechanism that makes your brain tell you to stop exercising when it begins to get tough, and the feeling of wanting to stop exercising only increases as you continue to push yourself harder to do more. This is all despite the biological fact that you are physically capable of doing much more than is being suggested by the messages you are receiving from yourself.

Over time, the brains of people who exercise regularly, especially at high intensity, will naturally adjust and reposition this built-in safety margin. This means that the brain of an experienced high-level athlete does not "tell" them to stop an exercise until the level of intensity is much higher than it would be for a beginner.

Therefore, how is it possible to subjectively quantify and then impart appropriate levels of recommended intensity when it comes to exercise? This problem is even more challenging when one considers that accurately translating and subjectively assessing various intensity levels will always be subjective to every individual.

If you were to train as hard as humanly possible, with near 100% maximum intensity, which involves super-strict form and training to complete failure and beyond, then you simply could not train for a long time. It is just physiologically impossible. Physics and biology are quite simple in this respect.

The intensity of your workout is directly proportional to the length of time you can physically perform it. The harder and more intensely you exercise, the shorter the time you can physically perform it.

Make no mistake, performing a 7-second isometric exercise while exerting close to your personal 100% maximum physical capacity is completely and utterly exhausting, even for a professional athlete.

What does all this mean when it comes to accurately communicating various levels of exercise intensity, especially when there is no professional coach or elaborate and expensive measuring equipment at hand?

Research clearly shows that almost everyone will stop exercising long before they are in any danger of becoming seriously fatigued. Most people will *think* they are exercising at a much higher intensity than they would if they were only a little more mentally resilient.

This does not mean that people should suddenly begin pushing themselves beyond their physical limits, which would be stupid. However, it does mean that most people who enjoy a higher-than-average level of mental resilience, determination, and being in physically good condition can push themselves much harder than they might think. If anyone ever feels "genuine" strain or fatigue to the point of becoming injured, then they should stop exercising immediately.

Even without the aid of a professional coach to monitor, encourage you, and measure your intensity and progress with specialist equipment, the tips we have outlined in this section will help you get the most out of every workout. It is also worth remembering that if you cheat, then the only person who loses is you.

As a footnote, for the sake of clarification, exercise intensity refers to how much energy is expended when exercising, including the amount of weight used per repetition. Perceived intensity varies with each person. Intensity and force are technically different, but are frequently accepted as interchangeable terms in the common vernacular.

Muscular strength is different from muscular endurance, which is the ability to produce and sustain muscle force over a certain period of time. While strength is the maximum force you can apply against a load, power is proportional to the speed at which you can explosively apply it. In other words, it is the ability to quickly produce a given amount of force.

Muscular force, often referred to as muscular strength, is the physical power exerted by muscles to perform various actions, such as lifting, pushing, or pulling objects. It results from the contraction of muscles and is vital for human mobility and functionality.

Technically, How Does a Muscle Grow?

How does a muscle grow? This is one of the most common questions concerning fitness and exercise. However, it is also one of the most misunderstood concepts, even amongst fitness professionals and personal trainers. To see for yourself just how uninformed or badly informed some people are, simply join one or two of the social media groups online so you can read some of the absolute drivel posted by 'keyboard warriors' who purport to be 'experts' on the subject. Alarmingly, many of these people seem to have developed a hardcore following, which to the science-based professional is like watching 'fools leading other fools' on a wild goose chase.

So, back to the key question, which is, how does a muscle grow? To explain this, we must examine three concepts: 1) muscle growth through increases in the volume/size of myofibrils inside the muscles, commonly called myofibrillar hypertrophy. 2) hyperplasia, which is when there is an increase in the number of muscle cells/fibres. 3) Sarcoplasmic growth, which is all about increasing the fluid content.

When it comes to exercise, the muscles you wish to grow must be challenged with a workload greater than they can currently accommodate. In other words, an exercise that is intense enough to stimulate growth. This stimulus can come from any source, such as lifting a heavy object, weight training, isometrics, compressing a spring in a device such as a Bullworker™, or through self-resistance, either hand-to-hand or limb-to-limb or using an Iso-Bow™, etc.

This process creates trauma to the muscle fibres, disrupting the muscle cell organelles. This then triggers other cells outside the muscle fibres to greatly increase in numbers at and around the point of the trauma to repair the damage. The process of repair involves a fusion of cells. This, in turn, causes the cross-sectional area of the muscle fibre to increase because the muscle cell myofibrils increase in both size and quantity. This process is more commonly known as hypertrophy. Since this process increases the number of cellular nuclei, the muscle fibres generate more myosin and actin. These are contractile protein myofilaments, which help make the muscle stronger.

This is the basis of what is more commonly known as myofibril muscle growth. In addition to this, there is also probably a process called hyperplasia. I use the term 'probably' because this concept is extremely controversial for many reasons. One of the key problems is that evidence of this in human beings is lacking, whereas there is a mass of evidence supporting hyperplasia in mice and other animals.

Hypertrophy is the increase in the size of the existing muscle fibres to accommodate the increased demands placed upon them through intense exercise. Hyperplasia, concerning skeletal muscle growth, is the increase in the number of muscle fibres, which in turn will also increase the cross-sectional area of a muscle.

Despite a lack of evidence supporting hyperplasia in human beings, logic supports the process. This is because of a theory known as Nuclear Domain Theory. This states that the nucleus of a cell (a muscle cell in this instance) is only able to control a finite area of cellular space. It is thought that satellite cells donate their nuclei to the muscle cell until a certain point is reached when this can no longer take place.

Beyond a certain limit, and through continued intense training, the cell must eventually divide to create two cells instead of the former single cell. When this happens, the entire hypertrophy process starts over once again. This probably means that most of the muscle growth is almost certainly caused by hypertrophy, and a much smaller percentage can be attributed to hyperplasia at any given point in the muscle stimulus/growth process.

Finally, the subject of sarcoplasmic muscle growth needs to be addressed. Sarcoplasmic muscle growth is the increase in the volume of sarcoplasmic fluid in the muscle cell. These fluids and energy resources surround the myofibrils in your muscles, containing mostly glycogen together with other elements, including creatine, ATP, and water.

To clarify, glycogen is simply a type of sugar that serves as a form of energy. It is deposited in bodily tissues as a store of carbohydrates, and it is the body's main form of storage for the sugar glucose. Glycogen is stored in two main places in the body, one being the liver and the other being the muscles.

More importantly, glycogen is the body's secondary source of long-term energy storage, with fat being the primary energy storage source. When glycogen is in the muscles, it is converted into glucose for use as energy when performing sports, etc., and glycogen stored in the liver is converted into glucose for use as energy throughout the body and in the central nervous system.

Therefore, sarcoplasmic growth increases muscle volume, but this increase is not in functional strength mass since it does not increase the number of muscle fibres. It is like 'the pump' in that it increases the size and shape of the muscle through the muscle holding an increased amount of fluid.

Rest Time Between Exercises

Naturally, the rest time between exercises during a workout is quite different from the rest and recovery needed to allow your body to respond positively to the stimulus generated by exercise.

If you keep the rest time between exercises brief enough, the workout routine itself will give you an excellent cardiovascular workout, and this is what we recommend that you ultimately aim for. If you are already very fit, we recommend that instead of performing the optional cardio routine, you simply put more effort, force, and intensity into each isometric exercise.

At the same time, aim to keep the rest time between those exercises as brief as possible. This approach will help you work towards performing each exercise with an Ultra-High Intensity Ultra-Short Burst™ effect, which will greatly improve your overall fitness level and boost your Base Metabolic Rate (BMR).

However, if you are not already fit, you may wish to begin by simply allowing each isometric exercise to deliver all the cardio you need as you gradually build up your fitness and endurance levels. This gradual approach ensures that you feel confident and reassured in your fitness journey. Eventually, you will increase your fitness level to a point where you can gradually reduce the rest time between each exercise to a minimum that works best for you.

Once you have learned how to fully engage the muscles during each exercise with sufficient force, and at the same time, you have learned how to breathe fully, deeply, and naturally throughout each exercise. At the same time, you should be keeping the rest time between exercises to a minimum because this combination will have an excellent and beneficial cardiovascular effect.

Dynamic Flexation™

Dynamic Flexation™ is a technique we devised to help ensure that we gain maximum benefit from the isometric portion of our exercise regimens. I will recap and briefly summarise the Dynamic Flexation™ technique as originally laid out in "The 70 Second Difference™" book.

We always recommend that everyone who performs any kind of resistance exercise practice some form of Dynamic Flexation™ before performing any exercise. This will help ensure that all muscles, tendons, ligaments, joints, and spine have become naturally and properly engaged in the correct biomechanical exercise position.

We would never recommend that you immediately apply maximum power and force as soon as you assume any exercise position. This is unless you are a very experienced athlete or unless you are training with a qualified coach to perform a certain type of isometric exercise to develop extra power, such as a static-dynamic or explosive/ballistic isometric technique. Instead, we recommend that you always breathe naturally as you gradually flex and engage your muscles and joints into performing the exercise.

To perform Dynamic Flexation™, you gradually flex your grip and the muscles you are about to exercise while applying an increasing level of force immediately before performing the exercise. The exercise is then performed, and to disengage from it, we recommend reversing the Dynamic Flexation™ engagement process.

We prefer to gradually apply tension and force to the exercise through Dynamic Flexation™, typically for between 2 and 3 seconds, or even for as long as 4 seconds if needed. This all takes place before beginning to count the required 7-second exercise time of the isometric contraction.

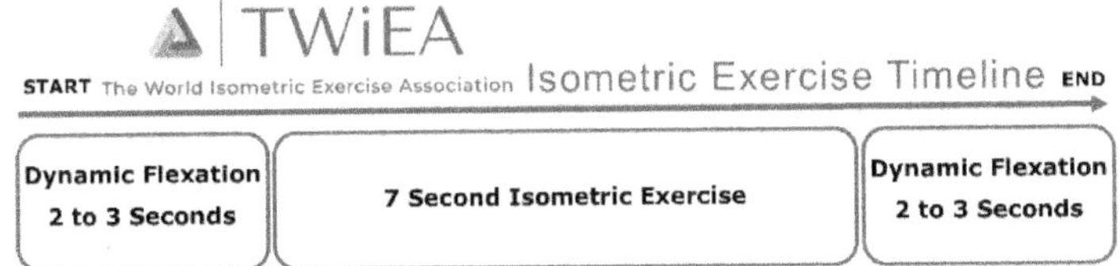

We prefer using one deep, full breath in and out to count each second that has elapsed more accurately. This way, you will time each exercise more accurately and not be tempted to hold your breath at any point, which is a mistake that beginners often make.

Similarly, at the end of an exercise, we do not recommend that it be ended abruptly. Instead, we recommend reversing the Dynamic Flexation™ technique so that you gradually relax as you slightly move each muscle and joint out of the exercise position.

This process helps enormously because when you are in a good position, you will gain the maximum benefit from each exercise you perform.

Dynamic Flexation™ is when you move and adjust your feet, legs, hips, and especially your hands as you gradually assume a solid position and handgrip. As you flex and move, you will be making micro-adjustments.

All exercises will be performed best if you assume a correct and solid handgrip, fist clench, or foot position, etc. One of the most important aspects of assuming the correct exercise position begins with your grip.

Without a solid grip on a bar, handle, or anything else you need to hold while exercising, you will naturally be setting yourself up to perform sub-maximally. You can also help develop injuries, which can include sore elbows, joints, ligaments, and tendons.

Dynamic Flexation™ is a concept that embraces the broader principles of motor unit recruitment and "Henneman's Size Principle" to increase the contractile strength of a muscle.

Elwood Henneman's principle stated that under load, the motor units in a muscle are engaged according to their magnitude of force output, from the smallest to the largest, and in task-appropriate order.

This means that the slow-twitch, low-force, fatigue-resistant muscle fibres are activated before any fast-twitch, high-force muscle fibres are engaged, which are less fatigue-resistant. Since the body naturally works in this way, it enables precise and finely controlled force to be delivered at all output levels.

This also means that fatigue will always be minimised when exercising or performing tasks in daily life. It will also be proportional to the sequential engagement of the most appropriate muscle fibres.

Isometric Exercises and Blood Pressure

Some exercise critics point out that performing an isometric exercise raises blood pressure. However, these people conveniently forget that the same is true of all other forms of exercise, including freehand callisthenics and traditional isotonic resistance training with weights.

ALL physical activity, especially exercise, will cause your blood pressure to rise for a short time. Providing that you are in good health, if you always breathe deeply, naturally and normally when performing any exercise, any rise in blood pressure will soon return to normal when the exercise stops. The faster this happens, the fitter you are.

For advanced athletes and/or those who have been used to hard and intense isometric training for a long time, you will already have made significant progress in strengthening your heart and circulatory system.

For those who are new to isometric training, just like with any form of exercise, the best way to get into it is by taking it slowly and less intensely at first. Newcomers to exercise, especially isometrics, should always focus on applying less force and breathing fully and deeply throughout all exercises. NEVER HOLD YOUR BREATH!

Under strict medical supervision, even those with Coronary Artery Disease and high blood pressure should be able to increase their physical activity levels with a reasonable degree of safety. However, if you already suffer from high blood pressure, you should always exercise at a much lower level of intensity than someone who has no physical issues.

FURTHERMORE, EVERYONE, ESPECIALLY PEOPLE WITH HYPERTENSION OR ANY FORM OF CARDIOVASCULAR DISEASE, SHOULD ALWAYS CHECK WITH THEIR DOCTOR BEFORE BEGINNING ANY KIND OF EXERCISE ROUTINE.

Rest and Recovery

Many factors must be considered when calculating your ideal recovery period. These include your age, current health and fitness level, the quantity of exercise you have done, and, most importantly, the intensity of the exercise.

Some people need a recovery period of between 24 and 48 hours; for others, it may be as brief as 12 to 24 hours. As a rule, the recovery period will always incrementally increase as the intensity of the exercises increases towards an individual's 100% potential maximum capacity. Always be aware of this, and make sure that you factor this into your rest and recovery time calculations. The diagram will help to outline this.

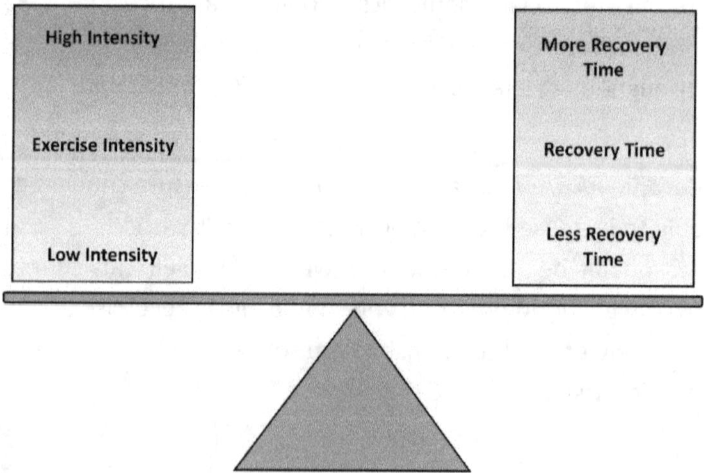

Sports scientist J. Atha's research revealed something remarkable. It showed that the average person could safely perform an exercise like this daily without overtraining when performing isometric contraction exercises at two-thirds of an individual's maximum capacity. Standard isometric contraction exercises can be safely performed daily by almost anyone of almost any age and in almost any physical condition as a means of strength development, body shaping, and even bodybuilding.

However, we recommend a full rest day between sessions for more intense workouts due to the higher demands placed upon the central nervous system (CNS) and the time needed to recover and fully benefit from the exercise. Several other factors affect post-exercise recovery. These include a balanced and properly executed stretching routine and getting enough quality sleep. While you sleep, your body releases certain hormones that help you repair and rebuild damaged tissue and will directly help your muscles grow.

Adequate Nutrition is Vital

Quality post-exercise nutrition will help your body repair itself faster, decrease your recovery time, and maximise the benefits gained from the exercise. Research shows that post-exercise immunodepression peaks if you exercise longer than you are currently capable, and problems are enhanced due to reduced or inadequate nutrition.

Hydration is also one of the most important factors in recovery and overall health, especially since muscles are mostly composed of water.

Early studies suggested a 30 to 60-minute window after exercise when you need to eat, after which your body begins to draw upon itself to repair and recover from your workout. Later studies found that this window can be anything from 1 to 3 hours, depending on the workout type, applied force, overall intensity, and goals. On average, since most leave 60 minutes after food before hard exercise, and if a workout lasts an average of 45 minutes, then a 30 to 45-minute window to eat after exercise will mean it has been up to 150 minutes (2.5 hours) since your last food; therefore, the earlier suggested 30–45-minute window still makes sense for most people especially if they want to build more muscle and strength.

Most people mistakenly consume excessive amounts of protein at the expense of other key nutrients, such as carbohydrates. Therefore, in doing this, they are working against their best interests and overall optimum health. One of the key nutrients that has been found to help enormously when in recovery from prolonged periods of heavy exercise is carbohydrates. A lot of research supports the hypothesis that carbohydrate is the most important nutritional factor in preventing post-exercise immunodepression. Most do not realise that the protein composition of human muscle is typically only somewhere in the region of between 18/9% and 21% protein (average 20%), and the rest is made up of water, glucose, lipids, and carbohydrates, etc. We will not go into more detail here; however, if you want to learn more about this and many other surprising nuggets of useful information about sensible nutrition and exercise, then they can be found in The 70 Second Difference book.

Strength, Stamina, Endurance, and Resilience

Understanding the difference between strength, stamina, and endurance is important because once you do, you will be able to devise the most suitable workout routines for your body type.

Muscular strength is possibly best understood as a muscle's capacity to exert force against resistance or weight. This is comparatively easy to measure because one's ability to lift a given amount of weight for a single repetition is a good measure of strength.

Stamina is the length of time at which a muscle or group of muscles can perform at or near their maximum capacity. For example, the number of squats you can perform with a given weight that is 90% of your maximum would be a measure of your stamina or the distance that you can carry a similarly heavy object, such as an anvil.

Endurance is all about time and your ability to perform a certain muscular action for a prolonged period, regardless of the intensity at which you are working.

Resilience is all about your ability to recover from whatever stresses and demands are placed on your muscles. However, resilience is mostly all about your state of mind, your mental toughness and ability to endure, perform and deliver under pressure, and how you recover quickly emotionally.

Your body's muscular composition will always determine your performance in certain sports. The amount of slow-twitch muscle fibres you possess will determine your performance at endurance-related events, and both type A and type B fast-twitch muscle fibres are all about explosive power and your ability to maintain it.

In simple terms, if you possess mostly slow-twitch muscle fibres, you will naturally be better suited to endurance sports. Alternatively, you are a natural weightlifter if you possess mostly fast-twitch muscle fibres.

It is important to note that no matter what your natural predisposition might be in this respect, with the correct training regimen, it is still possible to significantly increase your abilities in your naturally weaker opposing areas of speciality.

Biceps, Supination, and Strong Arms

When most people think about the biceps muscles, they only think about flexing the biceps and elbow joints to create a classic bodybuilder pose. However, there is a great deal more to the biceps muscles than this. While flexing the arm in the way I have just described might be a primary function, another equally primary function is the action of twisting the forearm and hand, otherwise known as supination. This is it in pictures.

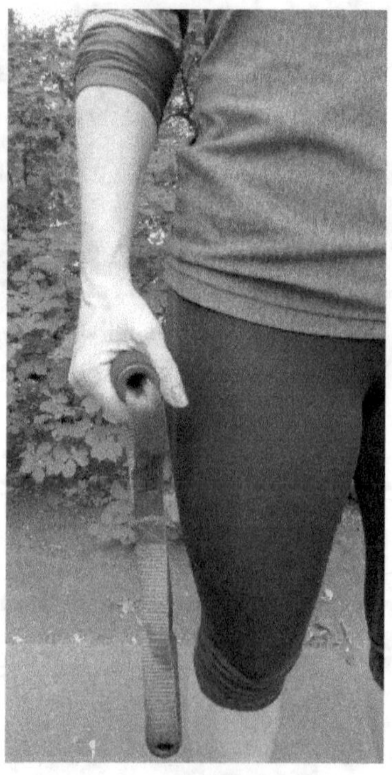

Neutral Position Front

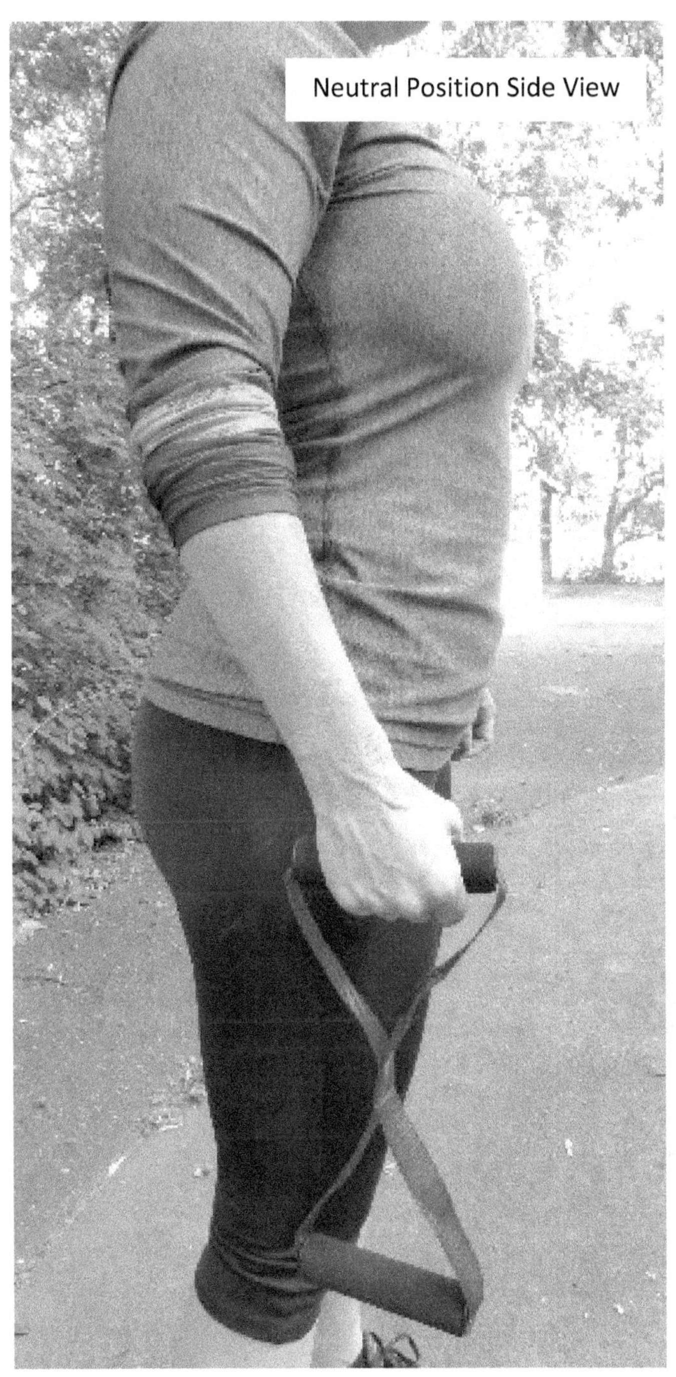

Neutral Position Side View

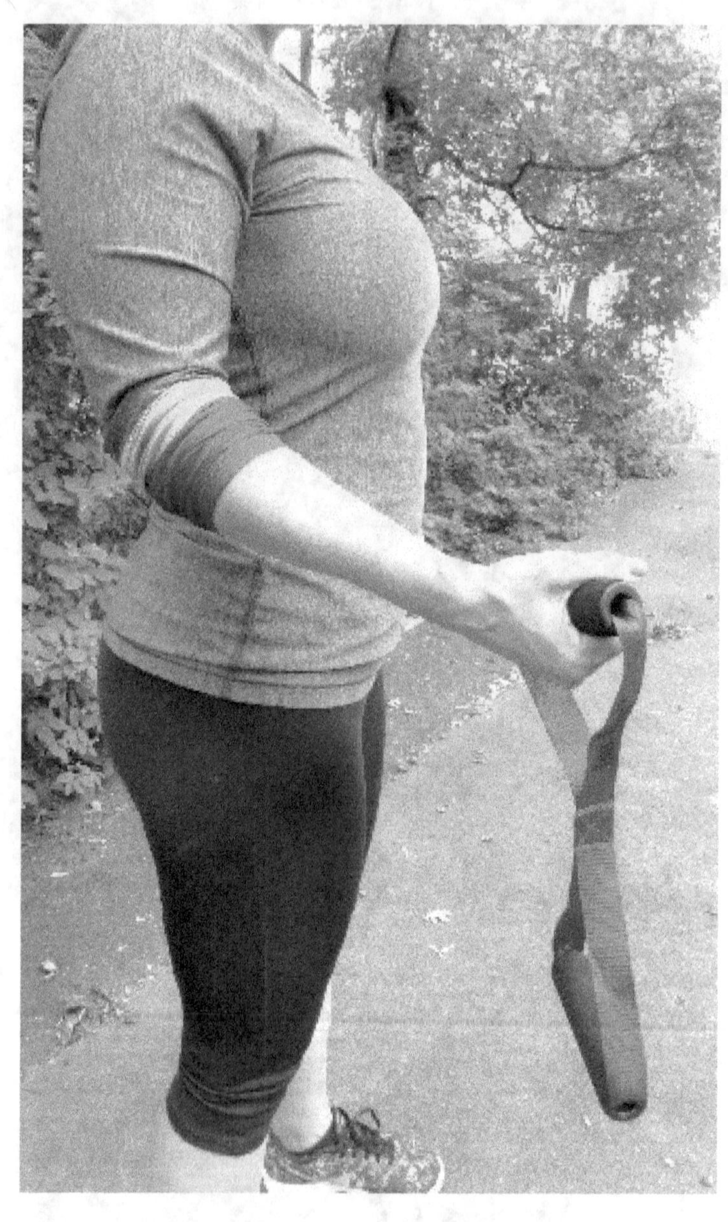

Mid Supination Side View

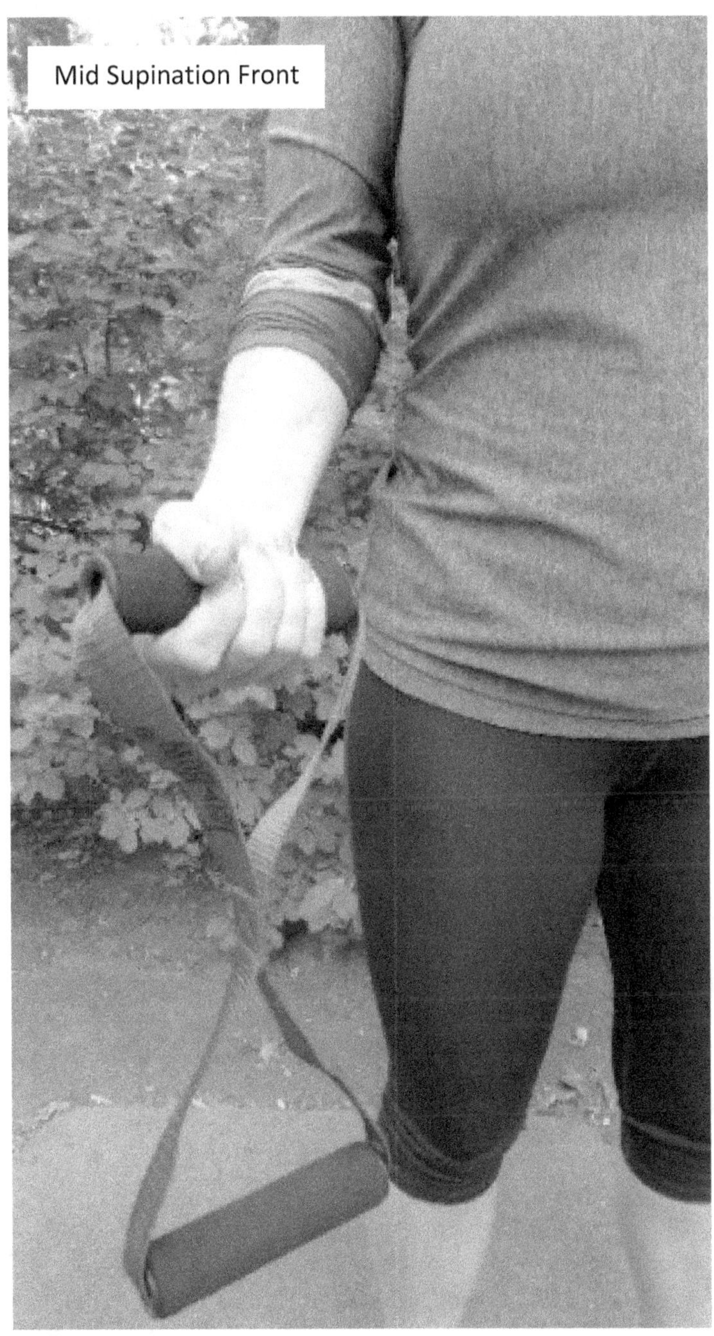

Mid Supination Front

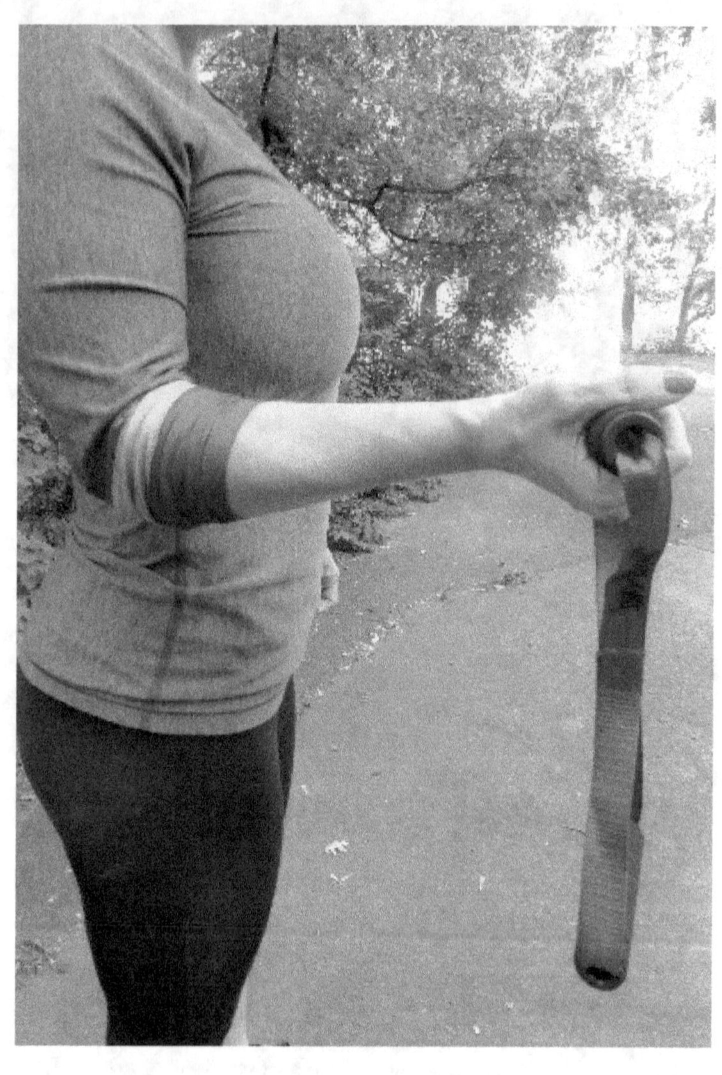

Full Supination Side

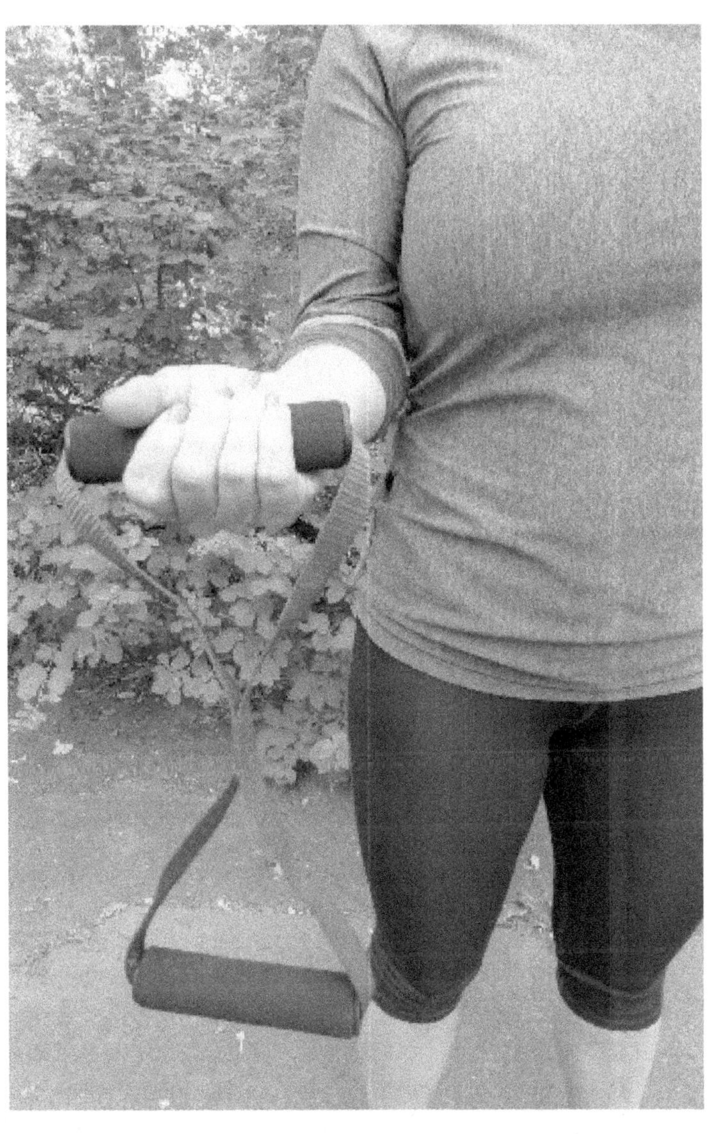

Full Supination Front View

Supination starts with the hand in a neutral position, roughly parallel to the side of your upper thigh. You twist it as you raise it until your palm is facing upwards at the top of the movement when the biceps are fully flexed. As most people think, the brachialis muscle is the primary mover of elbow flexion, not the biceps brachii.

This is because, even though the biceps brachii "show" muscle is seen flexed during a classic biceps pose, the brachialis that underlies it generates about 50% more power than the biceps brachii. Therefore, supination is important not only for elbow rotation but also for overall upper arm strength.

Therefore, you must consider all component muscles and their actions to gain maximum benefit and strength when exercising your overall front upper arm. The problem with isometric exercise in this respect, when pitting one limb against another limb or against a static, immovable object such as a wall, door or chair, is that it does not naturally allow the brachialis muscle to be exercised effectively. This is where the iso-Bow® fills the gap and enables a range of exercises to be performed in a neutral, partial, or fully supinated position.

- ▲ As a general rule, never allow your elbows to move forward or kick out to the side when performing a biceps curl.
- ▲ As with all curling exercises, never allow your wrist to bend backwards to fall out of alignment with the forearm because, in this position, you are between 3 and 4 times weaker than if your hand and wrist were locked in the correct biomechanical alignment.

Chapter 3: Other Potential IIEDs

One of the best things about isometric exercise is that if you do not want to use traditional gym equipment or proprietary devices, then you do not have to use them to perform a full workout. Instead, you can use nothing except your own body, immovable objects such as doors, walls, and door jambs, or readily available everyday items. These include walking sticks/poles, broom handles, towels, sturdy tow rope, or a climbing rope. I will list some of these items as suggestions for alternative equipment/devices for your workout sessions.

Improvised Isometric Exercise Devices
Rope – Either Climbing Rope or Towing Rope

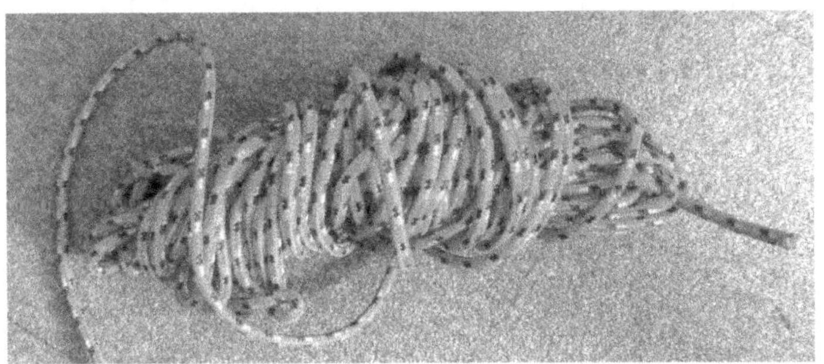

A rope is another simple but highly effective tool for performing an isometric and/or self-resisted workout routine. The important things to look for in a rope that might be suitable for exercise use are sufficient length, thick enough to allow a comfortable handgrip, and in good condition so that it will not break during your workout routine.

If you are using your feet to secure the rope, you may wish to loop the rope around the foot as shown for added safety and comfort. This will make it less likely to slip when it is pulled hard and more comfortable for the foot as well.

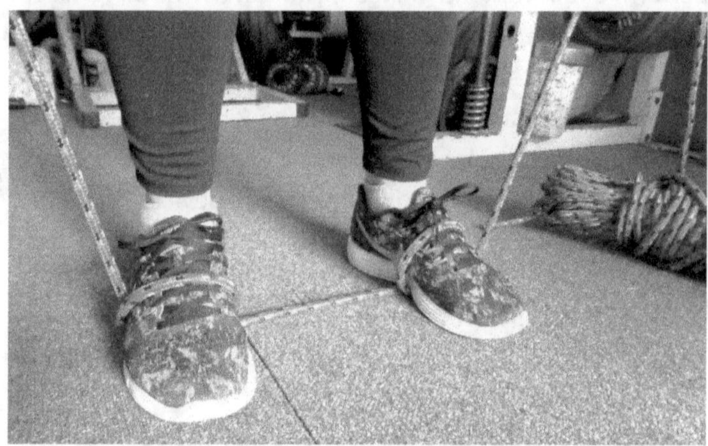

The Humble Beach or Bath Towel

The humble beach or bath towel is a common tool used by isometric enthusiasts who have nothing else to

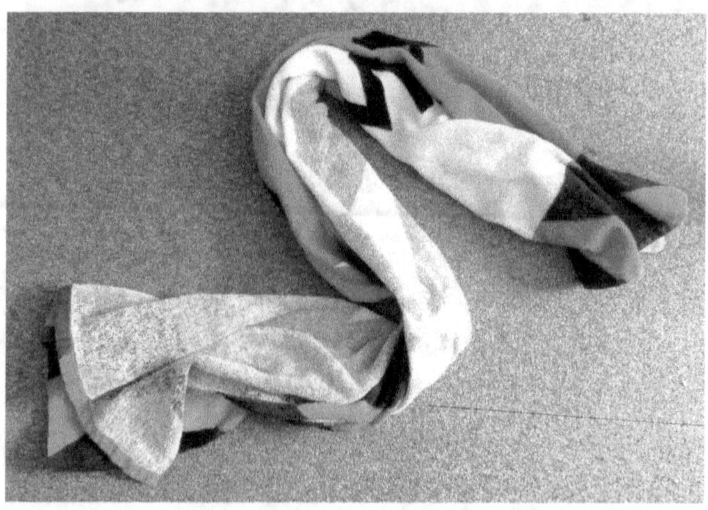

exercise with. It is also an exercise tool of choice for many because it is incredibly versatile. When choosing a towel to exercise with, the important things to look for are that it must be long enough and flexible enough to enable you to grip it properly, and therefore, it must not be too thick. Naturally, it must also be in good condition and not be liable to tear or rip during your exercise session.

The Broom Handle

The broom handle can be used almost identically to the walking stick or pro-style walking pole. By its very nature, it is not nearly as flexible as a walking stick or pro-style walking pole. This is because you can easily take a walking stick or pro-style walking pole virtually anywhere because that is precisely what they have been designed for. You would appear very odd indeed if you were to carry around a broom with you to exercise, whereas a walking stick or pro-style walking pole would not look even the slightest bit out of place. If you use a broom handle at

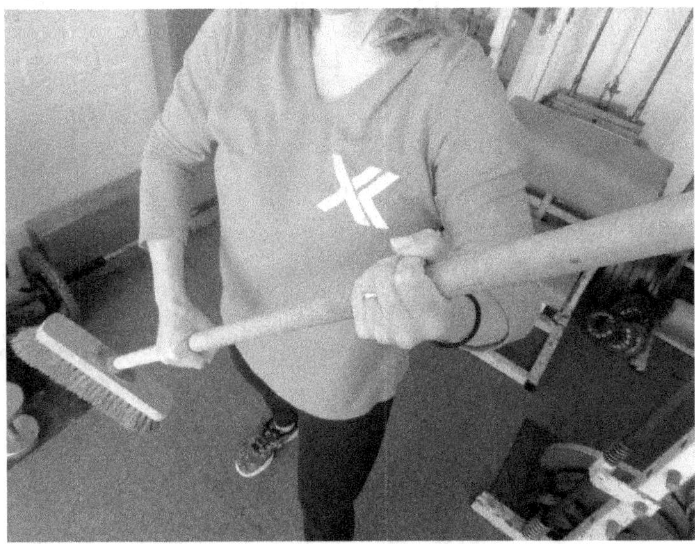

home to exercise with, then make sure it is solid and will not break when used in a workout routine. Also, we would strongly caution against using one to support your body weight in any way, with the broom handle to support it.

The Walking Stick/Pole

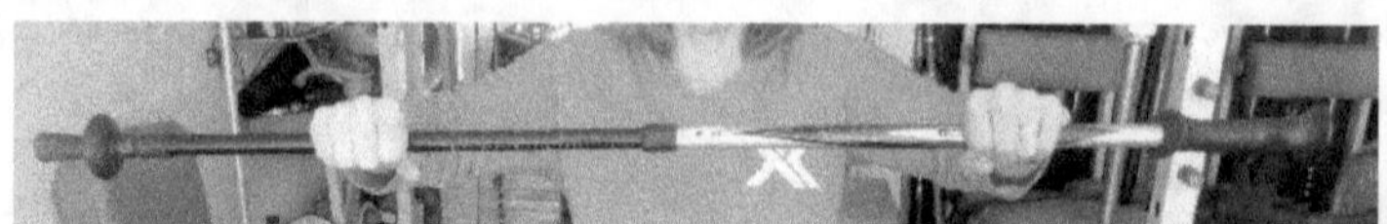

The walking stick or pro-style walking pole is an excellent device to use for an isometric workout. It is an improvised equivalent of a barbell or Bullworker® Classic without the steel cables on each side. One of the great advantages of the pro-style walking pole is that it can be adjusted to various lengths, making it easily adaptable for use in various exercises.

Many of the exercises can be performed alone without any need for partner assistance. If a workout partner is available, an even greater range of exercises can be performed. Nordic Walking Poles are different from ordinary walking poles, but they work equally well for isometric exercises.

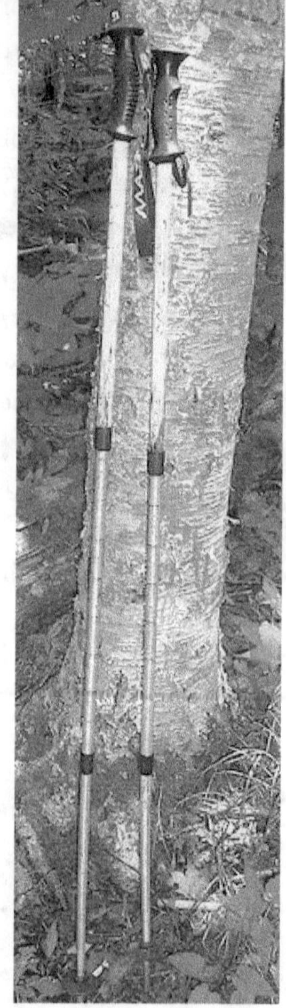

Photo: Daniel Case

Proprietary Isometric Exercise Equipment

We highly recommend and endorse the Iso-Bow®. as an exercise tool. This inexpensive little device is amazingly versatile and allows self-resisted isometric, isotonic, and functional isokinetic exercises to be performed easily. The Iso-Bow® provides the user with a biomechanically sound grip handle, which allows almost all exercises to be performed more effectively and with greater ease and comfort.

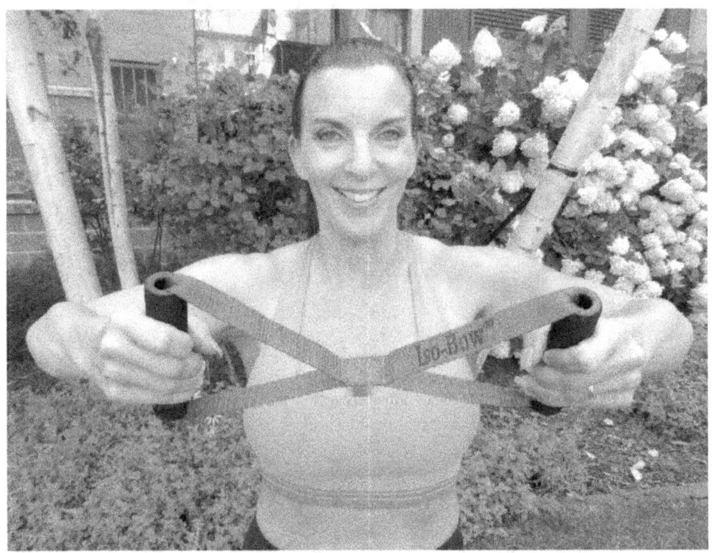

With a pair of Iso-Bows®, you can effectively exercise every major muscle group of the body and even perform advanced exercises such as pull-ups, the isometric squat, and the isometric deadlift. The level of workout you can get from using a pair of Iso-Bows® can range from an easy, low-level beginner's workout right up to a very high-intensity professional athlete level of workout. Amazingly, you can do all of this without any adjustment being needed to the Iso-Bows®. Each user will benefit proportionately, according to the amount of effort, force, and intensity that is applied during each exercise.

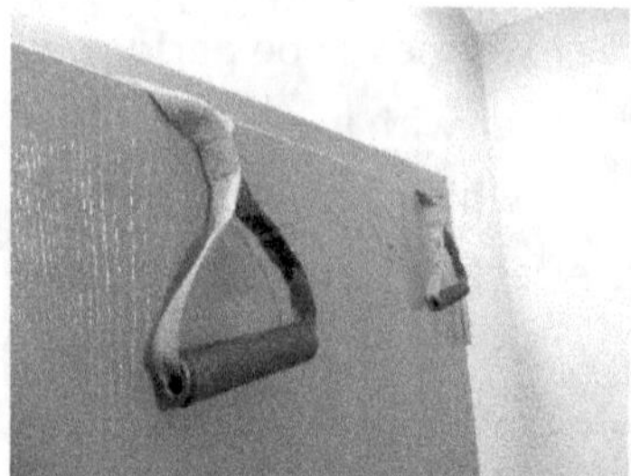
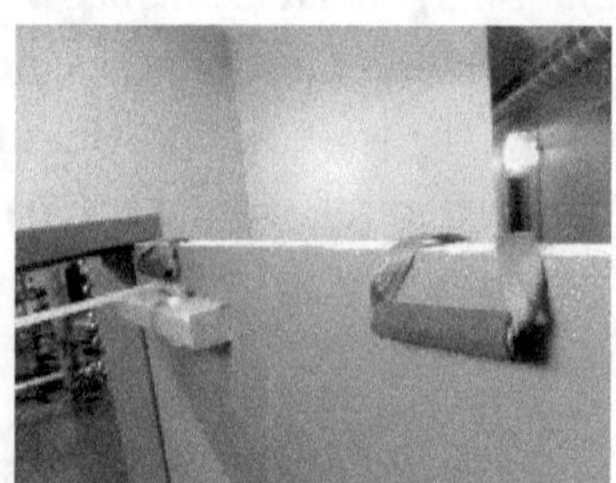

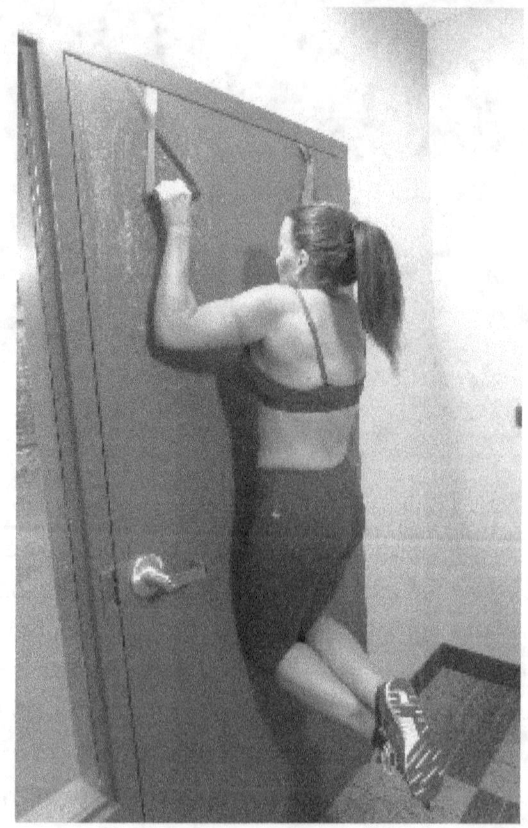

One of the standout features of the Iso-Bow® is its portability. It's so compact that it can easily fit into your pocket, handbag, briefcase, or backpack. This means you can take your workout with you wherever you go, making it the perfect companion for your busy lifestyle.

Perhaps the best-known of all isometric/isotonic home exercise devices is the Bullworker®, which has been a best-seller since its launch in the early 1960s. Today, it is still a best-selling device, and with good reason: It works. The smaller "partner" device is called the Steel Bow®, and both have interchangeable springs so that men and women of all strength levels and abilities can use them with roughly equal effectiveness.

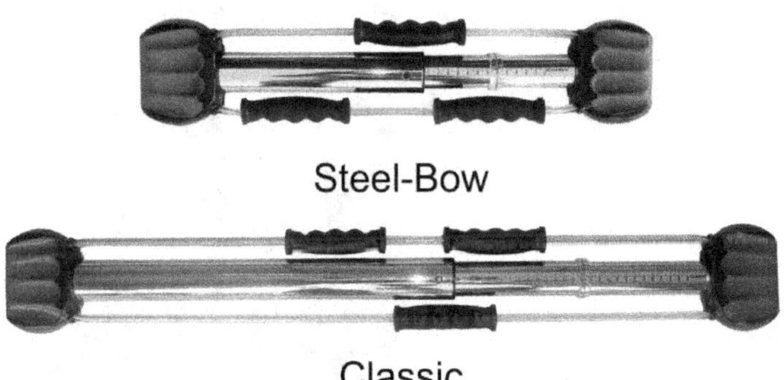

Steel-Bow

Classic

Securing the Iso-Bow® With Your Feet

When performing leg exercises such as squats and lunges, as well as lower back and glute exercises such as the deadlift, it becomes necessary to secure the Iso-Bow® using your feet properly. There are several ways in which the Iso-Bow® can be secured using your feet, and your preference of how you do this will depend upon many factors, such as your foot size, choice of footwear, and ease of operation.

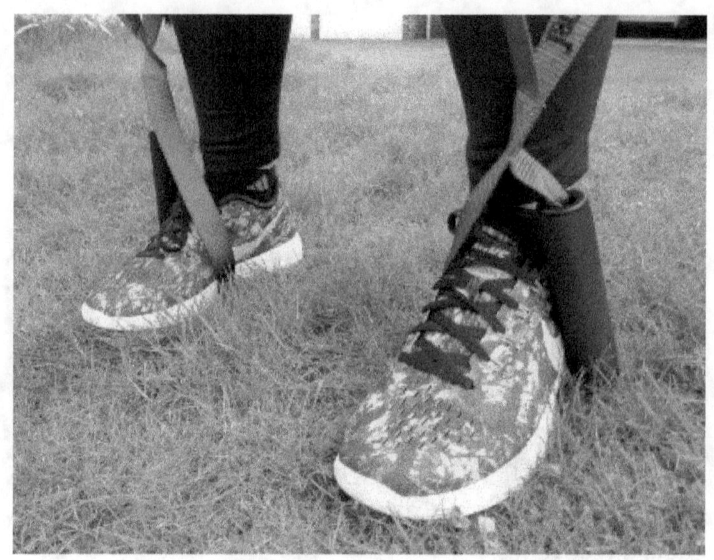

You can secure the Iso-Bow® with your foot inside one of the handles. To do this, adjust the handgrip to one side, usually the foot's outer side, and then place your feet inside the loop like a stirrup. Another method is to place the Iso-Bow® flat on the floor and then stand on one side of the straps so that the handle of the same side sits flush with your inner foot. In this position, your bodyweight combined with the handle pressing against the inner side of your foot enables you to pull safely and securely.

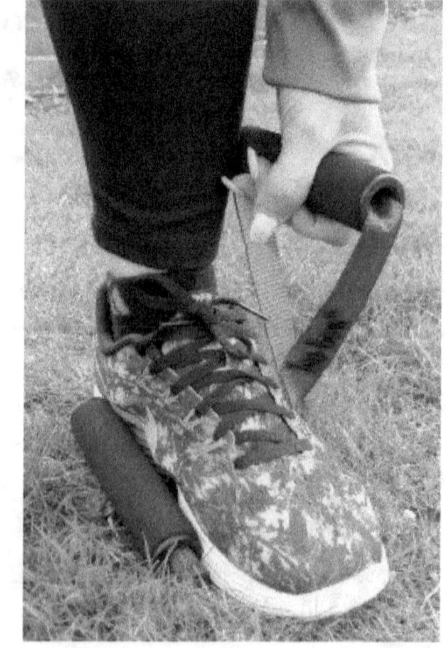

71

The final method is to simply place each foot through one end of an Iso-Bow®, stepping onto the foam hand grip as you do so. This method is slightly less stable than the other two methods. However, if the foot can be pushed far enough through the loop of the Iso-Bow® handle, then the handle will slightly raise the level of your heel, making it easier for some people to squat or lunge.

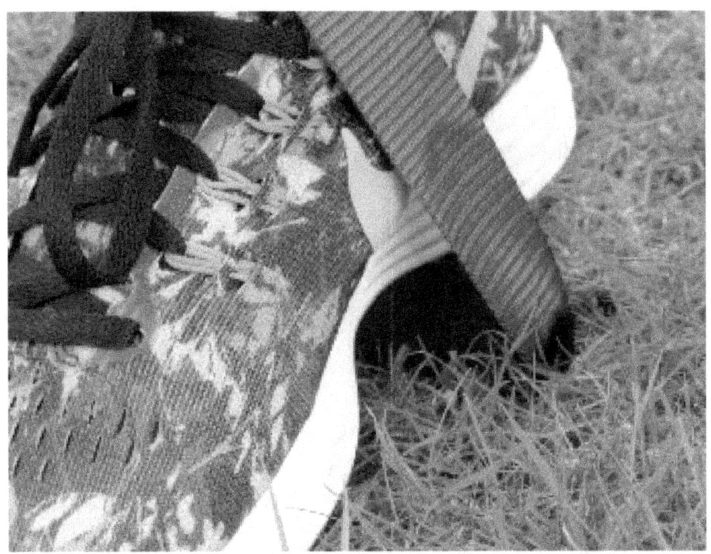

Naturally, safety is always a top priority, so whichever method you ultimately choose to use, always make sure that when securing the Iso-Bow® with your feet, there is never any chance of it slipping while you exercise.

Shortening The Iso-Bow® - The Cradle

Generally, the Iso-Bow® is the ideal size for most people to use with each exercise. However, occasionally, you may prefer to reduce its operational size by roughly half by creating what we call an Iso-Bow® cradle. To do this, place

72

one of the handles inside the webbing loop of the other handle side of the device. The webbing then cradles the handle you have just placed inside the loop and can be gripped as normal. Your thumb and fingers can then wrap around the foam handle and the cradle loop's webbing to help create an even firmer grip position.

This reduced size allows for an even greater operational range within the movement capability of each limb/joint to be created for certain exercises. These include the Cross-Chest Press, the Upper Back Power Pull, and the Biceps and Triceps Cradle Press-Curl.

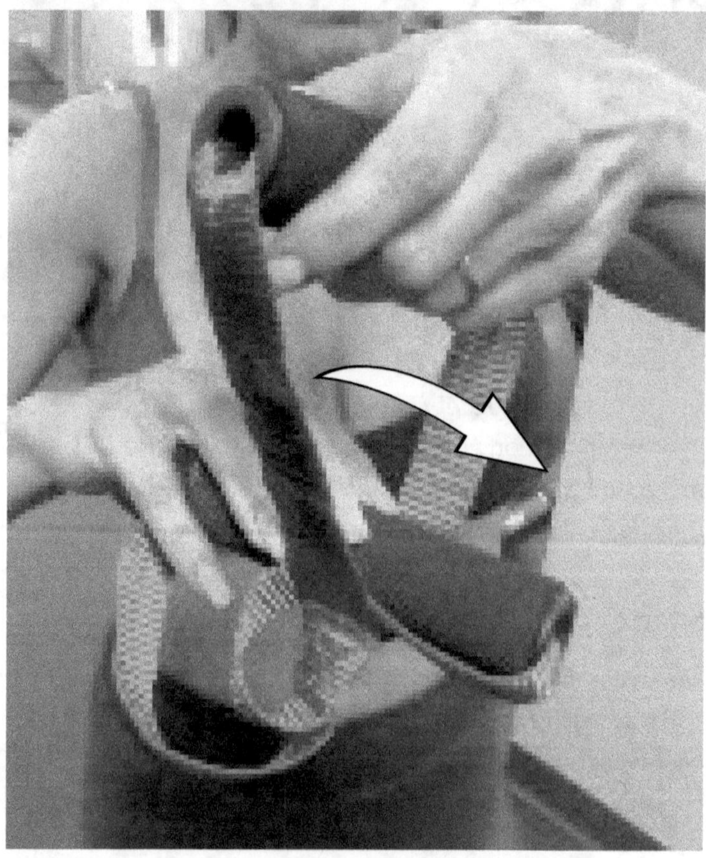

Chapter 4: About the Exercise Model

Helen Renée is originally from Duluth, Minnesota. She has lived in various locations, including North Pole, Alaska, where her father worked as an Ice Road Trucker, and then for a short time in Minneapolis before settling in Manchester, England. She is the author of 39 books to date and has achieved best-selling status on Amazon's top-10 list three times.

Helen is an isometric exercise instructor and a champion Bikini Fitness Athlete who achieved spectacular contest-winning results after embracing the isometric and trisometric exercise systems.

To achieve this success, she went from being almost 50 lbs overweight to a contest-winning condition in less than six months as a plant-based athlete who uses science-based workout sessions lasting no longer than 10 minutes per day.

She exercises daily, and when she is training to enter a contest, she always applies progressively more force than a normal person who simply wants to get a little stronger and fitter and maintain a good overall body shape.

Together with her husband, Brian, she was a consultant for the National Health Service (NHS) research and innovation department, providing specialist training in advanced isometric exercises as part of their Workout at Work program.

She is a Reiki Master Teacher registered with the Federation of Holistic Therapists and has authored a comprehensive six-book series on Usui Reiki, covering all levels and specialities, including animal Reiki.

Helen is a gifted Tarot master reader who has designed and published several sets of Tarot cards, all embracing the time-honoured Rider-Waite tradition. In her spare time, Helen enjoys researching and attempting to solve mysteries. She co-founded the unique Paranormal Rescue.com research and investigation team.

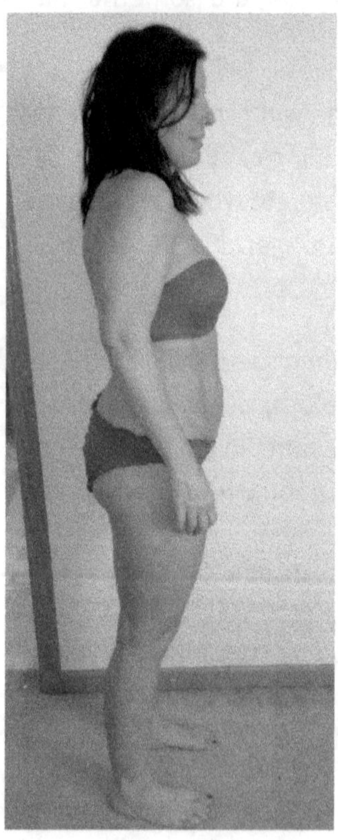
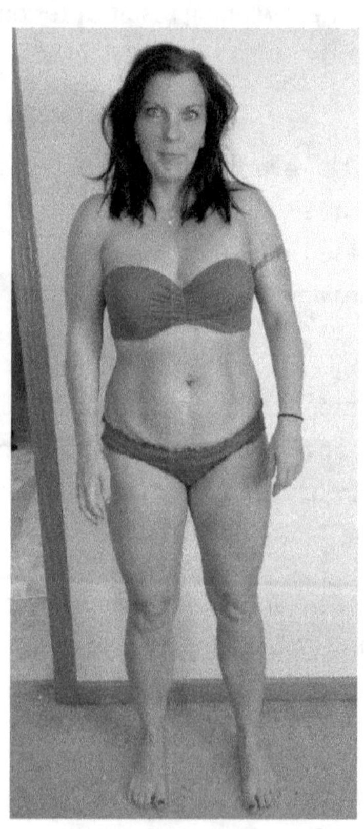

Her latest book on the subject, Quantum
Paranormal—Quantum Physics Explaining Paranormal
Phenomena, is the result of her collaboration with her
husband. Helen's notable contributions to paranormal
research have attracted extensive media attention, with
appearances on ITV's This Morning, BBC News, and Beast
Seekers, and coverage in publications including The Sun,
The Daily Mail, The Daily Mirror, Chat Magazine, Newsweek,
Forbes, and The Reader's Digest. To learn more about
Helen, visit www.HelenRenee.com

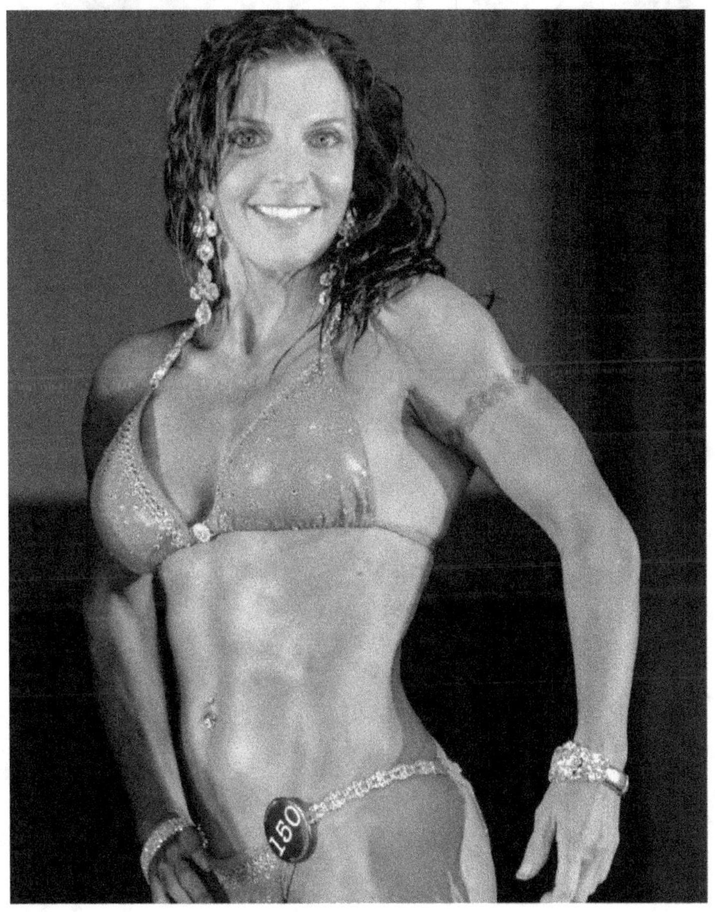

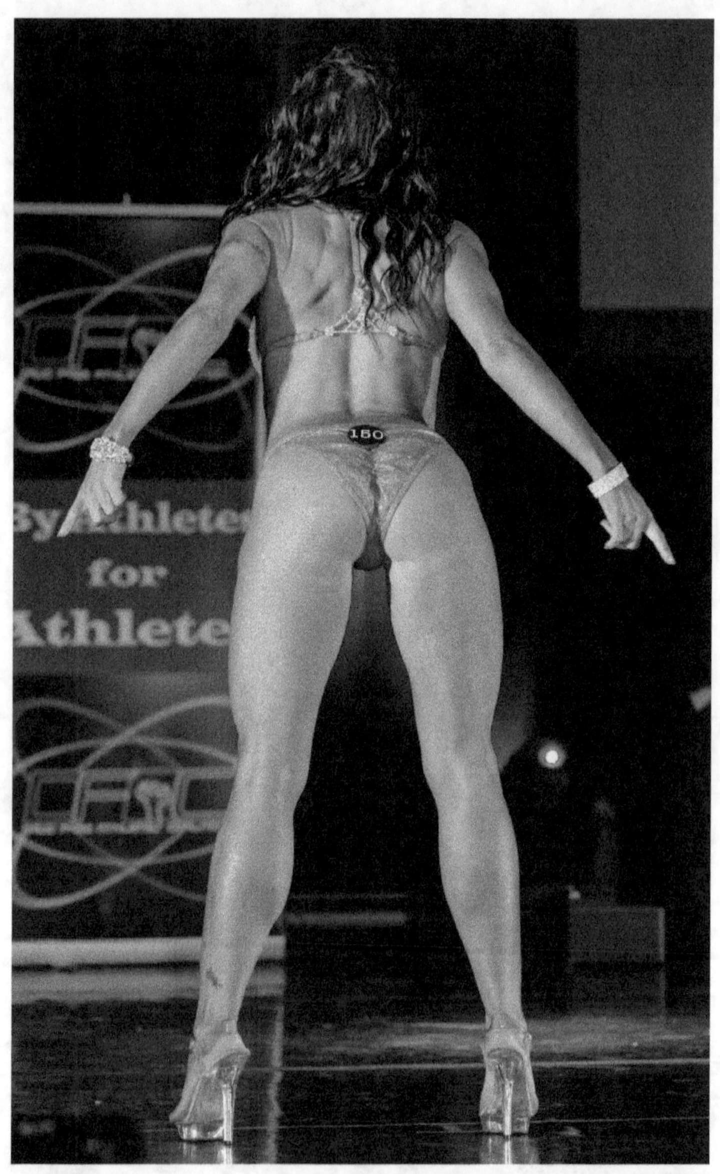
By Athletes
for
Athletes
150

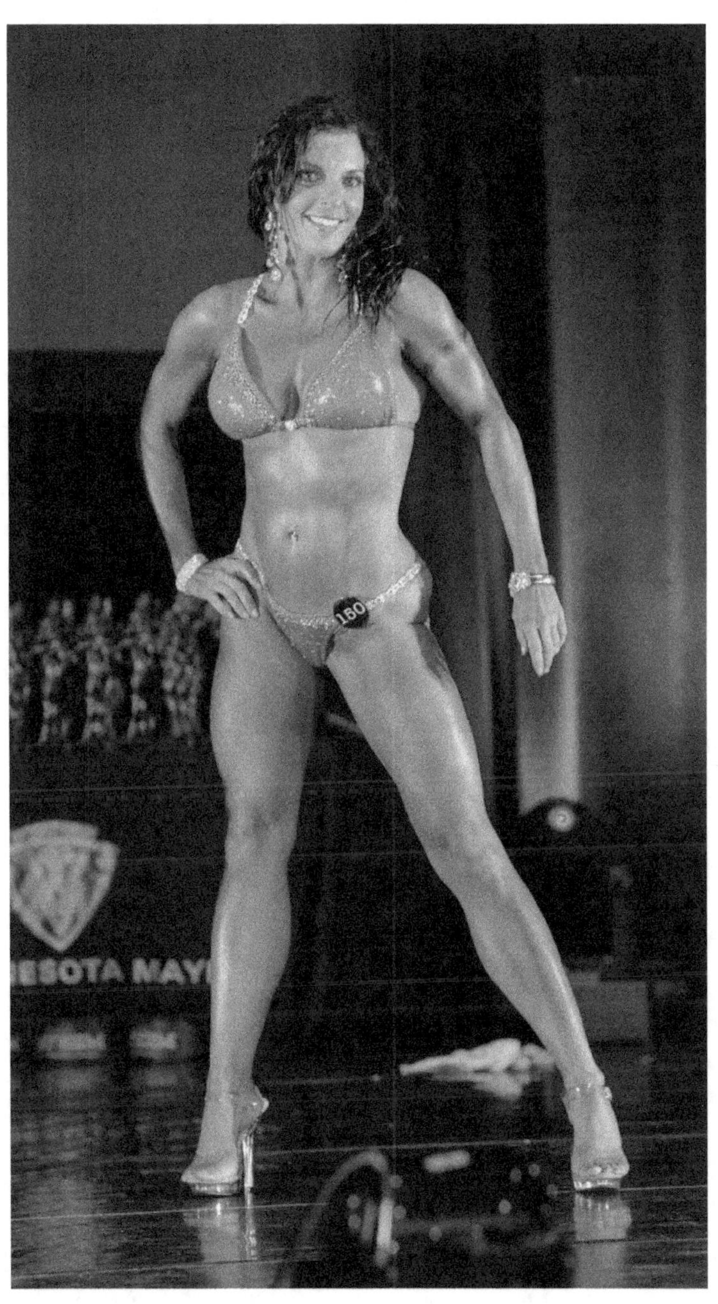

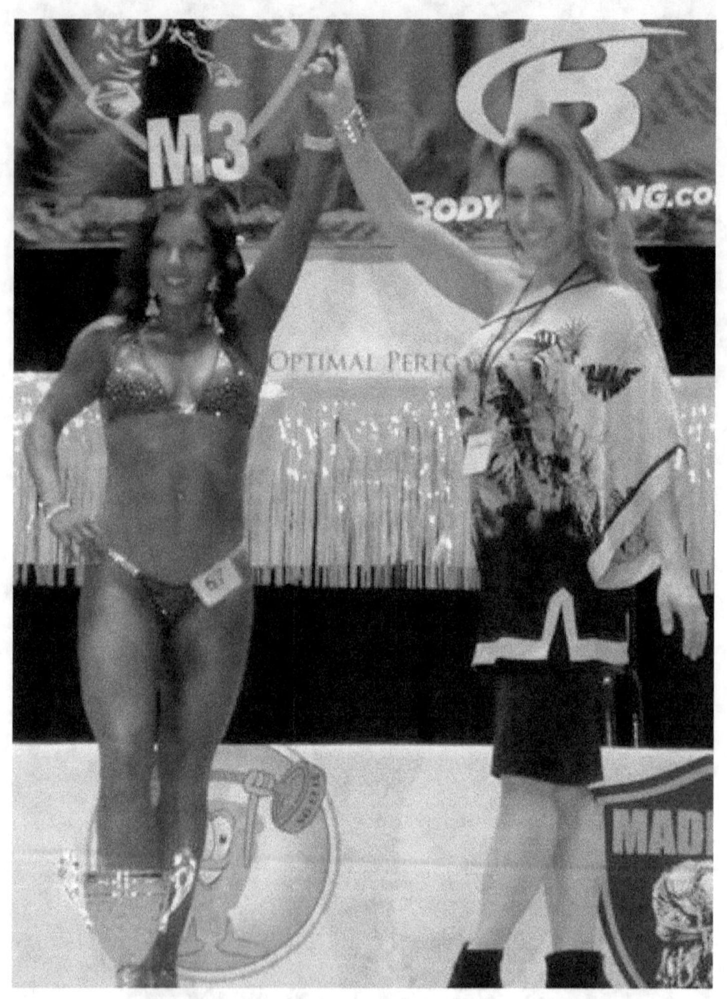

M3
BODY...ING.co...
...OPTIMAL PERFOR...
MAD...

The Author and an Isometric Experiment

The following picture is of my arm, taken in December 2016. It is the result of a year-long experiment to see what results could be gained through a basic high-intensity isometric exercise routine using only the minimum number of exercises.

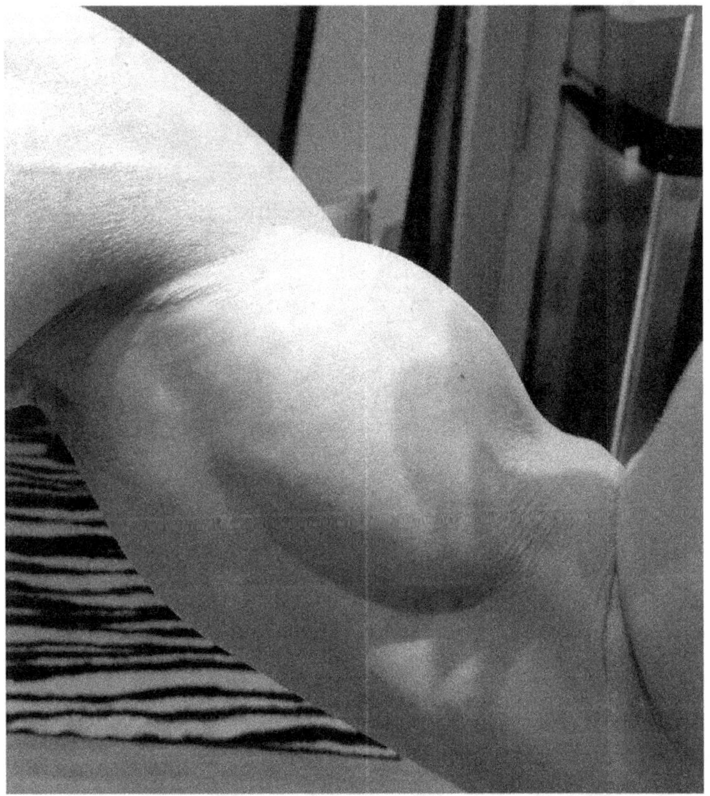

My arm after 1 year of basic isometric maintenance training. This picture was taken to record the results of the experiment in December 2016.
The routine allowed just 1 x 7-second isometric exercise per muscle/muscle group per day at a target level of applied force/intensity of between 75% and 80%.

For one year, starting in January 2016, I performed a daily 10-exercise x 7-second total-body isometric routine. It is common for even the most experienced athletes to count the elapsed exercise time increasingly quickly, almost in direct proportion to an increasing level of applied force/intensity. Therefore, I typically aimed to perform a 10-second isometric hold for each exercise, and this way, I would always reach the desired goal of 7 seconds in good style.

My target level of force for each exercise was around 75-80%, slightly higher than the typically recommended average of two-thirds or 66.6%. However, this still effectively meant that I exercised each of my biceps for a total of between just 21 and 30 seconds per week, nothing more.

Amazingly, at the end of the year-long experiment, I achieved an improvement in both the strength and size of each arm, albeit slightly. Even though I am well-versed in the science of isometrics, I still found it remarkable because it was in exchange for a maximum of 30 seconds per week of exercise time. Once again, this only reinforced that the best results are always gained through pinpoint focus, high intensity, and never confusing activity with accomplishment.

Chapter 5:
Things to Remember Before You Begin

- ▲ The first and perhaps the most important thing to remember is: **NEVER HOLD YOUR BREATH AT ANY TIME.**
- ▲ Breathing in and out naturally during all isometric exercises will also help you count the number of elapsed seconds much more accurately, with one full breath in and out taking approximately one second.
- ▲ We recommend that you read the instructions about each exercise carefully.
- ▲ Always leave a safe distance between you and others if exercising with any proprietary device or IIED (Improvised Isometric Exercise Device)
- ▲ Always check the structural integrity of any type of exercise device. If there is any doubt about the structural integrity, then do not use it for exercise or any other purpose.
- ▲ Before use, double-check that all adjustable joints on the exercise device and/or IIED are secure.
- ▲ Weight loss/fat loss will ONLY occur when any exercise plan is used in conjunction with a calorie-controlled diet.
- ▲ It is critically important to focus your mind on the exercise being performed completely. Envision the muscle you are exercising growing larger and stronger.
- ▲ Always consult a professional coach to devise a detailed stretching routine; this will ensure that you

are stretching the areas effectively rather than risking injury.

- ▲ Always ensure that a stable line of biomechanical progression is achieved before engaging in and performing any exercise.
- ▲ Warming-up, stretching, and cooling down are three of the most overlooked yet essential elements of exercise, and we cannot stress their importance strongly enough.
- ▲ During ANY form of physical exercise, including isometrics, if you apply too much force too soon, then you may inadvertently strain a muscle. Isometric exercise is particularly intense, and a single isometric exercise engages many more muscle fibres than even high-intensity weight training and at a much higher level.

For safety's sake, we always recommend using Dynamic Flexation™ to gradually and progressively engage your muscles in ANY exercise, especially isometrics, according to what we call The ISOfitness Exercise Engagement Timeline™.

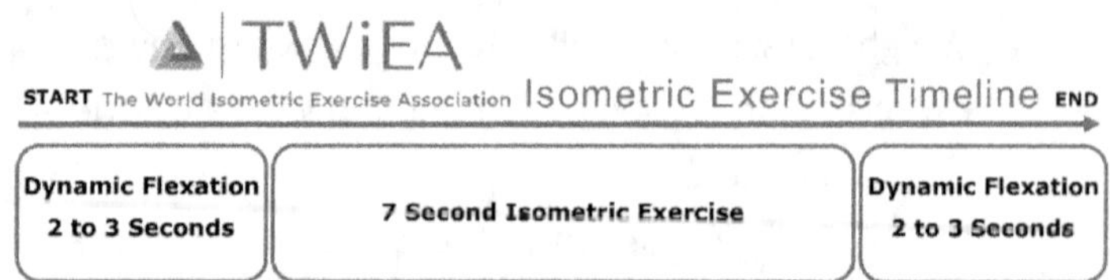

The main benefit of properly warming up for several minutes before a workout is injury prevention and increasing your heart rate and circulation to your muscles, ligaments, and tendons. It is important to remember that warming-up and stretching are two different concepts and that stretching is not a good warm-up. This is because

83

stretching will put the muscle in an uncontracted position and weaken it. Stretching is always best performed after a workout has been completed, together with a proper cool-down. In addition to properly warming-up, always perform a gentle flex and stretch of the muscles and joints that are about to be exercised. For example, squatting down fully to flex the thighs and loosen the knees is always a good idea before performing any leg exercises. Dynamic Flexation™ performed before any exercise should help to ensure greater flexibility and increased blood supply to the muscles and surrounding tissue.

Isometric exercises are deceptively powerful. Even when engaging in what may feel like only moderate-intensity exercise, you are probably still engaging and contracting many more muscle fibres than you would in a similar isotonic exercise. If you have any doubts, always perform the exercise with less force. All exercises and workout plans work equally well for men and women, and both can build strength, muscle, body build, or simply get into great shape, each according to their natural ability.

In our exercise resource books, the exercises listed are suggestions of what can be performed for each body part/muscle group. We do not suggest that they all be performed. Instead, users may wish to select the most suitable exercises from each section. In our course books, please perform the exercises according to the workout session notes. **Finally, please reread and review the 'Important General Safety and Health Guidelines' section to ensure that you have fully complied with all recommendations. Only start using the isometric or any exercise system with the full approval of your physician.**

Connecting Daisy Chains

As we know, daisy chains come in two or three standard variations of similar length. However, they all have interconnected loops, which make them ideal IIEDs. They can also be easily linked with a carabiner and looped with climbers' slings.

All daisy chains have a foot loop at one end and either a screamer (webbing link) or a standard loop at the other. This makes it easy to interconnect them to other daisy chains, carabiners, or the foot loops of other daisy chains. Therefore, with a pair of daisy chains and a couple of climbers' slings and carabiners, you have a comprehensive IIED toolkit.

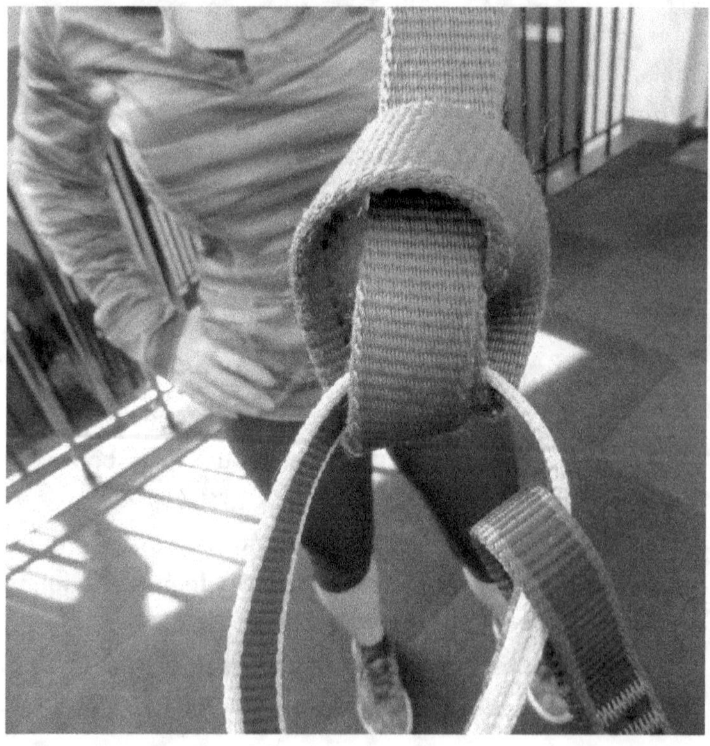

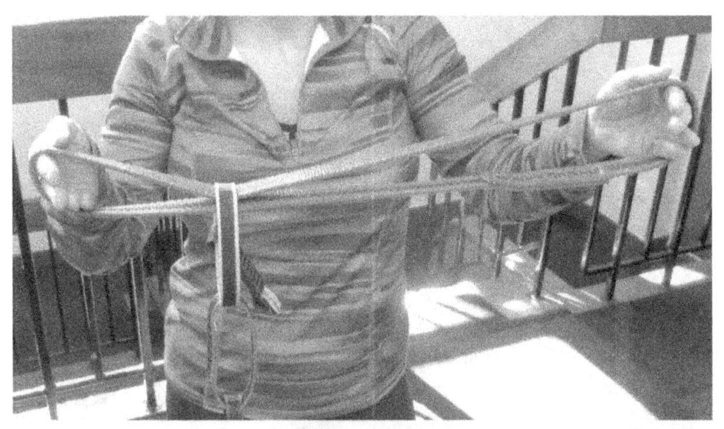

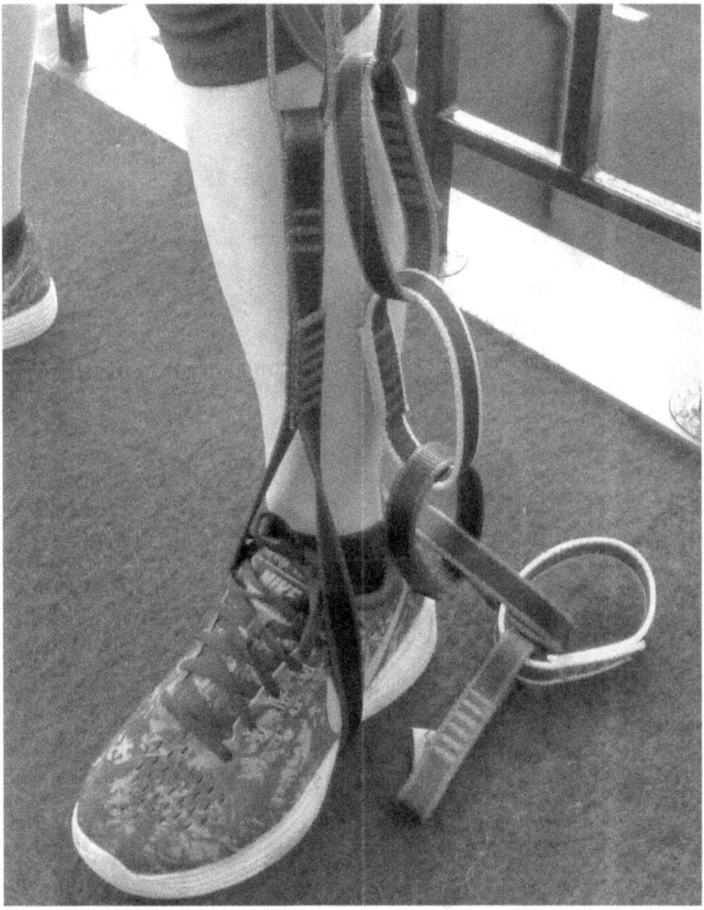

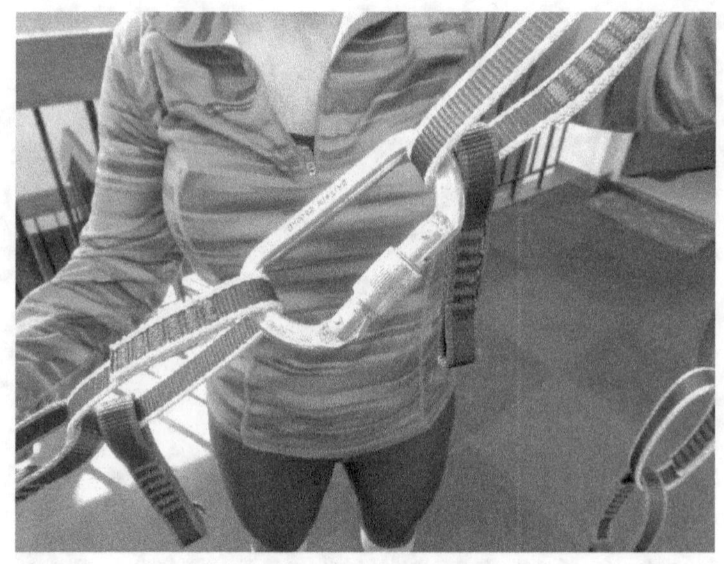

ABOVE: A DAISY CHAIN LINKED BY CARABINER

BELOW: A DAISY CHAIN LINKED BY SCREAMER AKA WEBBING STRAP

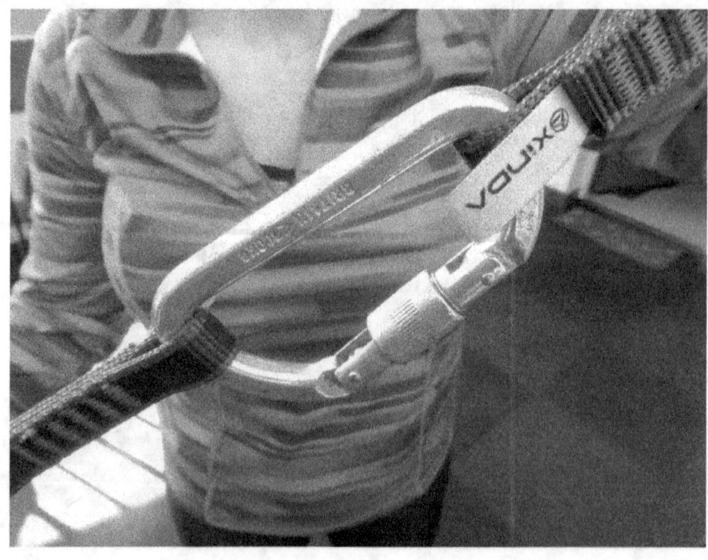

Chapter 6: Exercise Resources

Section 1 Abdominals:
Knee Raise and Trunk Curl

Sit on a chair or any other solid object and place the daisy chain face downwards over the top of one knee. Then, curl your body forward and downwards by contracting the abdominals, and at the same time, raise the knee, resisted by the daisy chain. Perform the same exercise on the other leg if desired.

When you perform an isometric exercise, never hold your breath. Always breathe deeply and naturally, which will be about 10 full breaths in and out at a rate of about 1 second per full breath. Perform each exercise for no less than 7 seconds and no longer than 10.

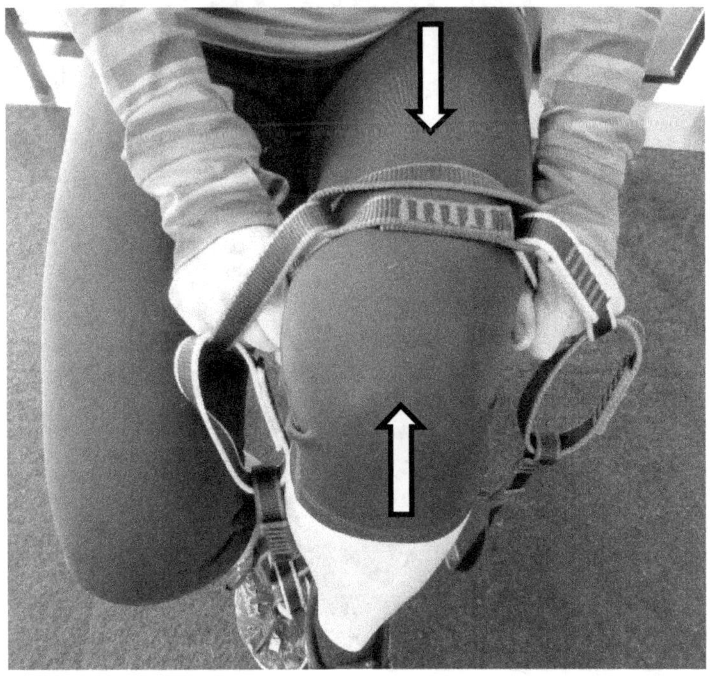

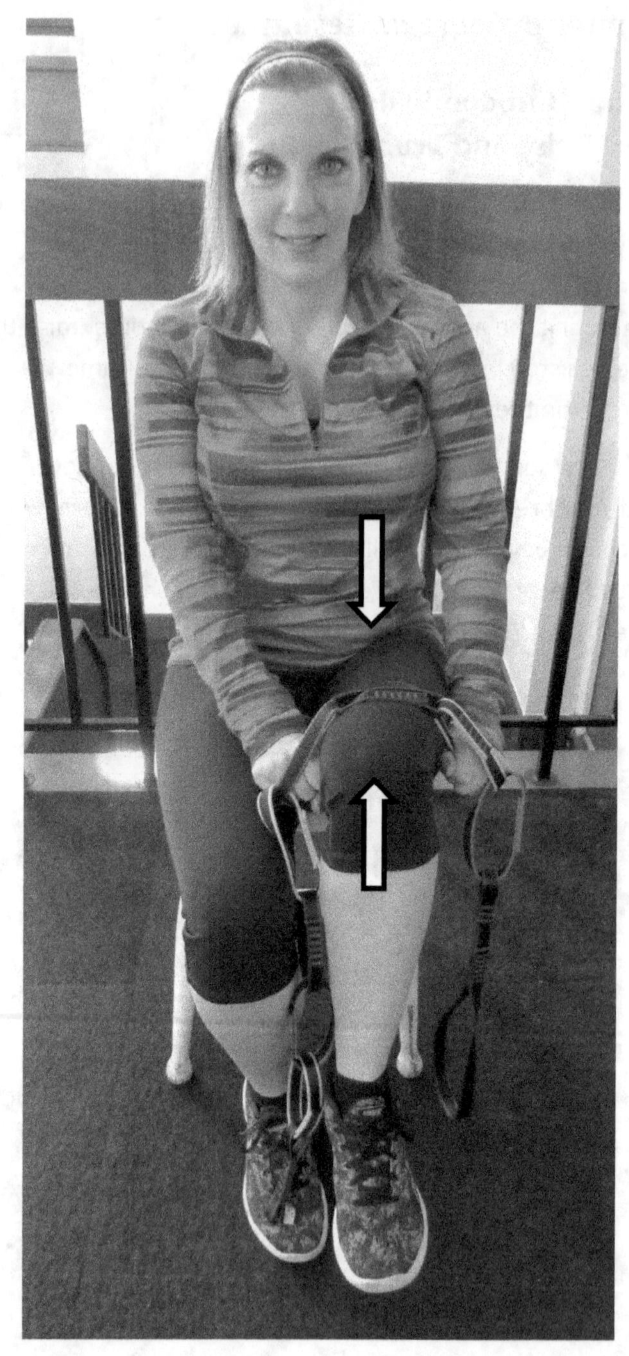

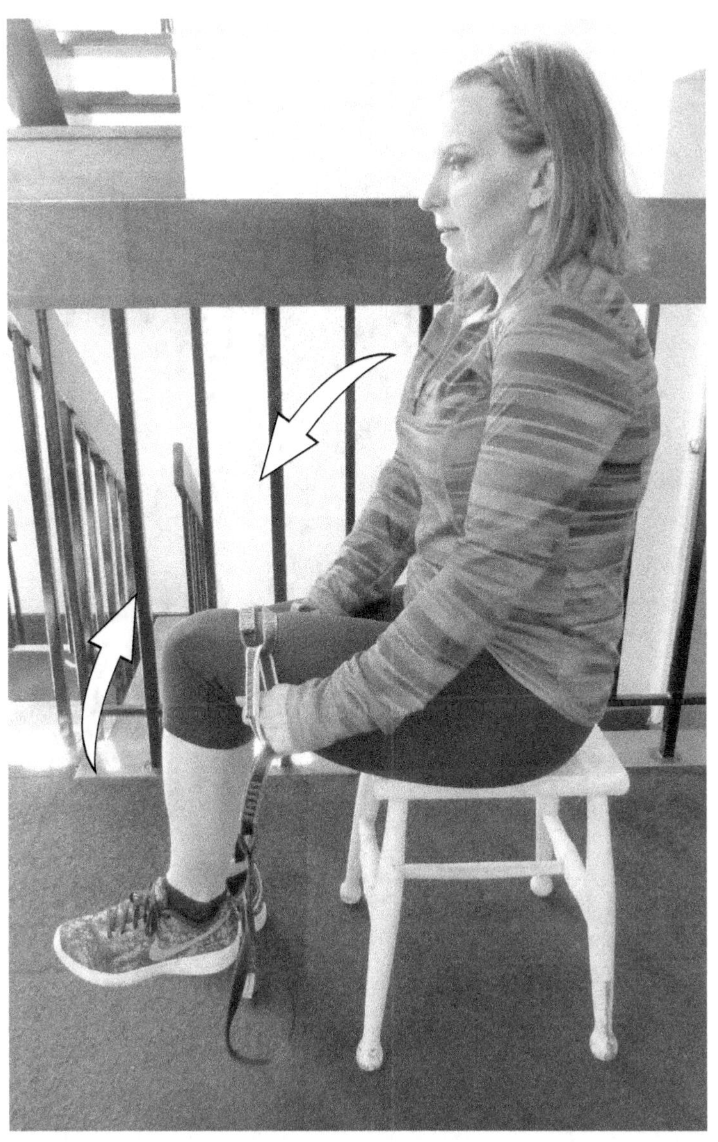

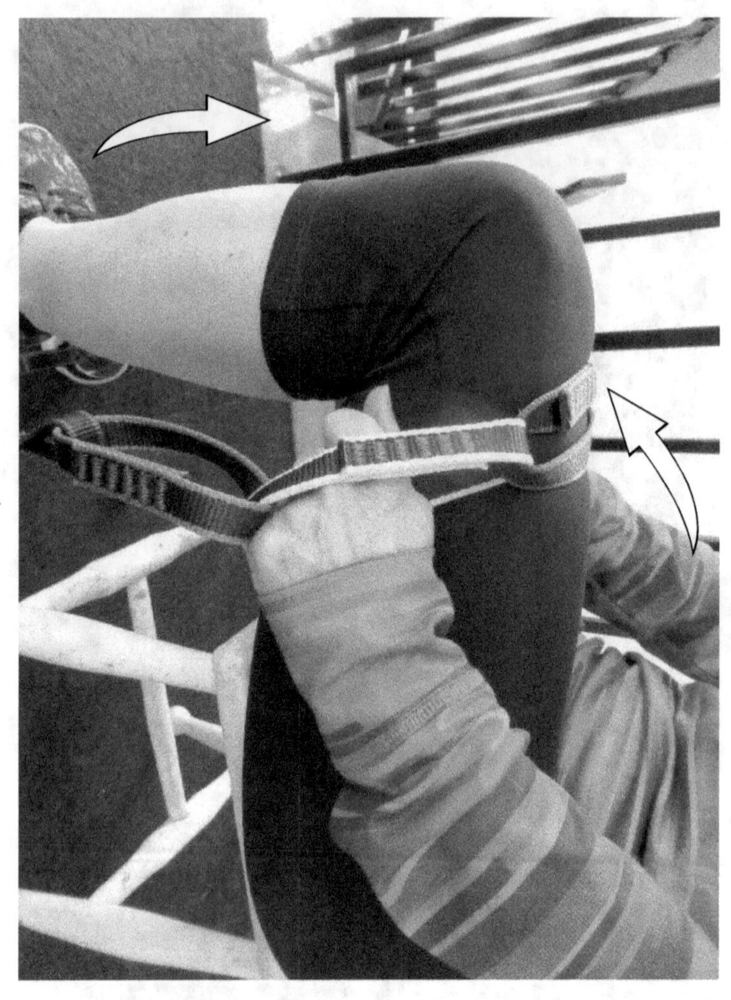

Section 1 Abdominals:
Trunk Curl Lying

Sit on the floor and find something solid and heavy to support your feet underneath. Bend the knees to an angle of about 90 degrees. Take a daisy chain in both hands and curl your torso upwards using the abdominal muscles. When you have reached a position with your shoulders slightly off the floor, engage the climbing sling to push against the front upper thighs just above the knees. In this position, use the abdominal muscles to try and raise the torso higher while, at the same time, you are being prevented from doing so by pressing the daisy chain against your knees/thighs.

When you perform an isometric exercise, never hold your breath. Always breathe deeply and naturally, which will be about 10 full breaths in and out at a rate of about 1 second per full breath. Perform each exercise for no less than 7 seconds and no longer than 10.

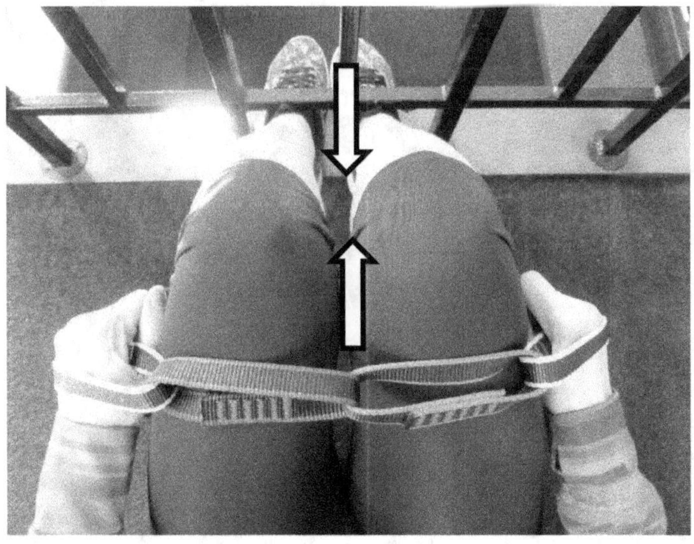

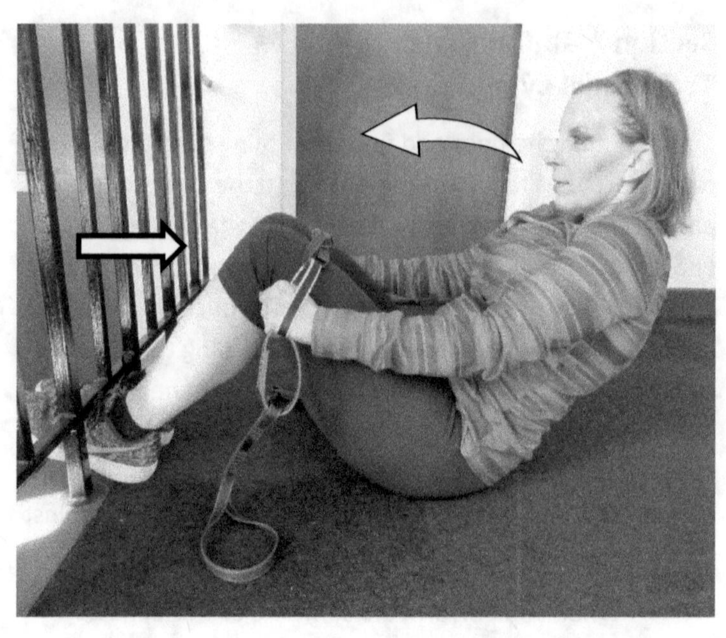

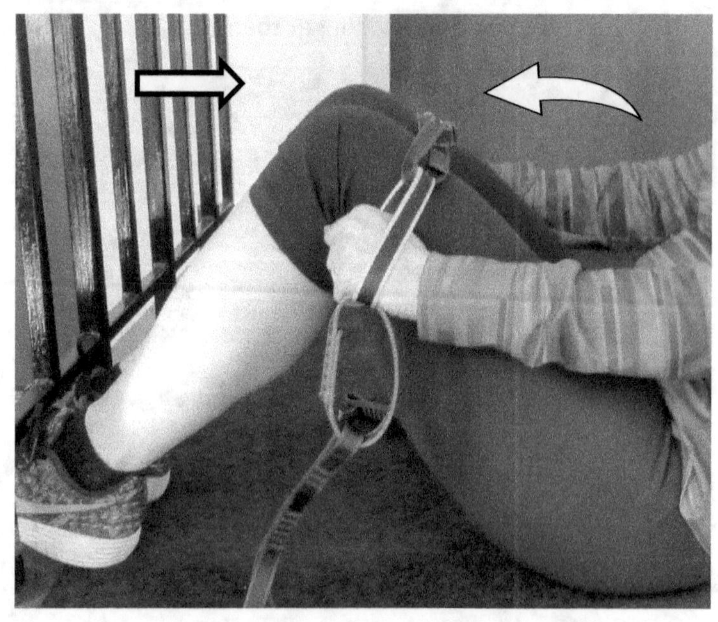

Section 1 Abdominals:
The Side Bend

Stand upright with your knees slightly soft and your hips aligned in neutral, facing forward, together with your torso. Place the foot loop of a daisy chain under one foot. Bend sideways as far as possible without allowing your hips to shift sideways or in any direction out of neutral. Take hold of a loop of the daisy chain at that level. Then, engage the abdominal oblique muscles on the opposite side of your body. Use these muscles to drive the action as you attempt to raise your torso sideways and upwards, back into the upright position again. When you have reached the desired level of force, then perform the exercise. When you perform an isometric exercise, never hold your breath. Always breathe deeply and naturally, which will be about 10 full breaths in and out at a rate of about 1 second per full breath. Perform each exercise for no less than 7 seconds and no longer than 10.

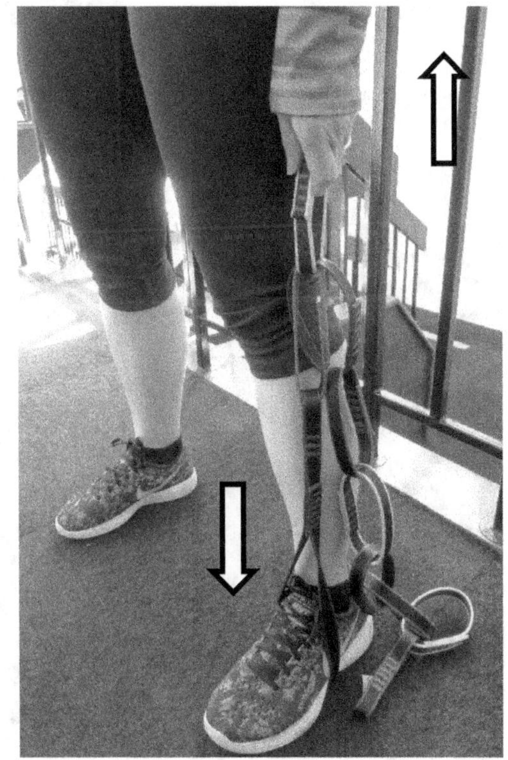

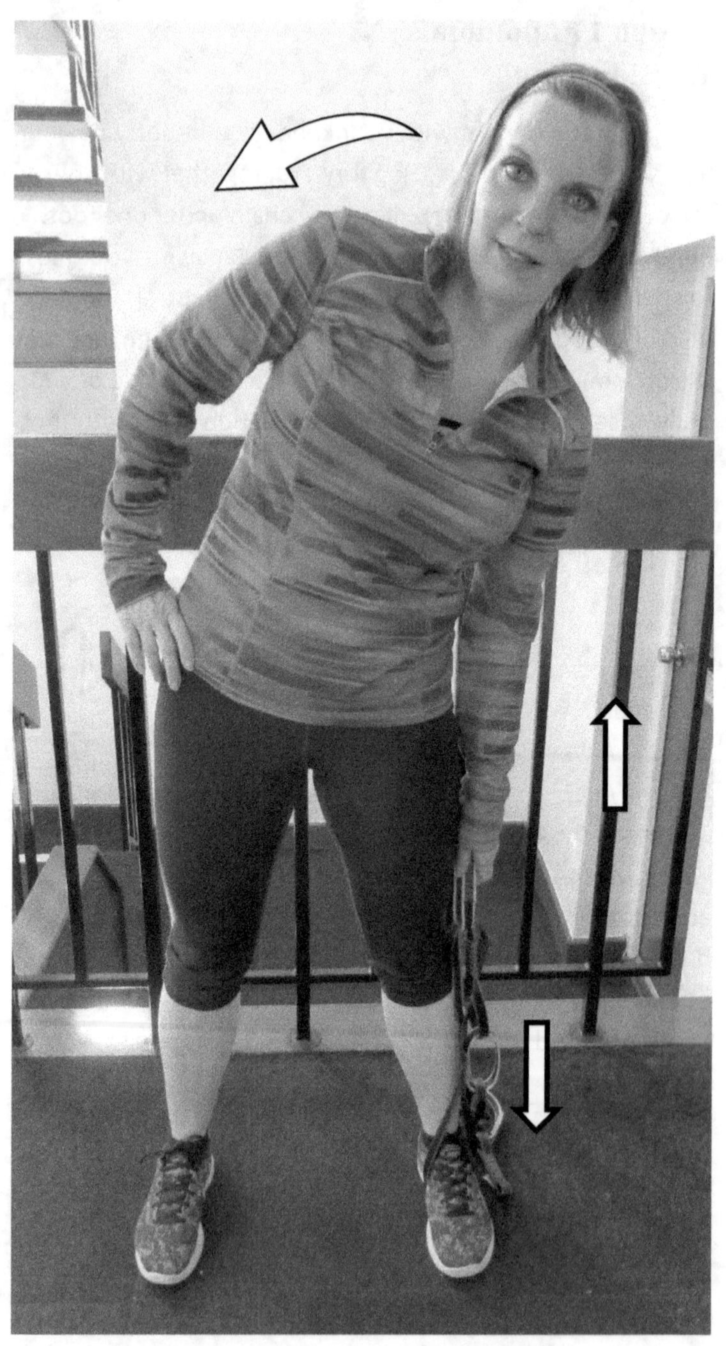

Section 2 Biceps:
Biceps Curl Kneeling (Both Arms)

Kneel on the floor with one foot forward, as shown in the pictures. Place the foot loop of two daisy chains around the forward foot. Keeping your torso upright and facing forward, take hold of a loop of each daisy chain in each hand. Choose the same colour to make it easier, and for general exercise, select a loop that allows the arm to curl to an approximate mid-point position, as shown. Keep your elbows back and engage the biceps muscles of each arm as you attempt to perform a biceps curl. When you perform an isometric exercise, never hold your breath. Always breathe deeply and naturally, which will be about 10 full breaths at a rate of about 1 second per breath. Perform each exercise for no less than 7 seconds and no longer than 10.

Note: If you use a single daisy chain, remember to exercise both arms/sides. Advanced users can perform the exercise using different loop positions to exercise the biceps muscles at different angles on the ROM, or Range of Motion.

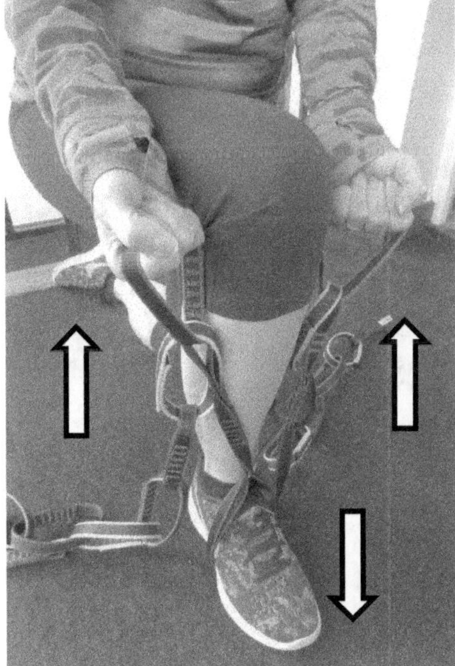

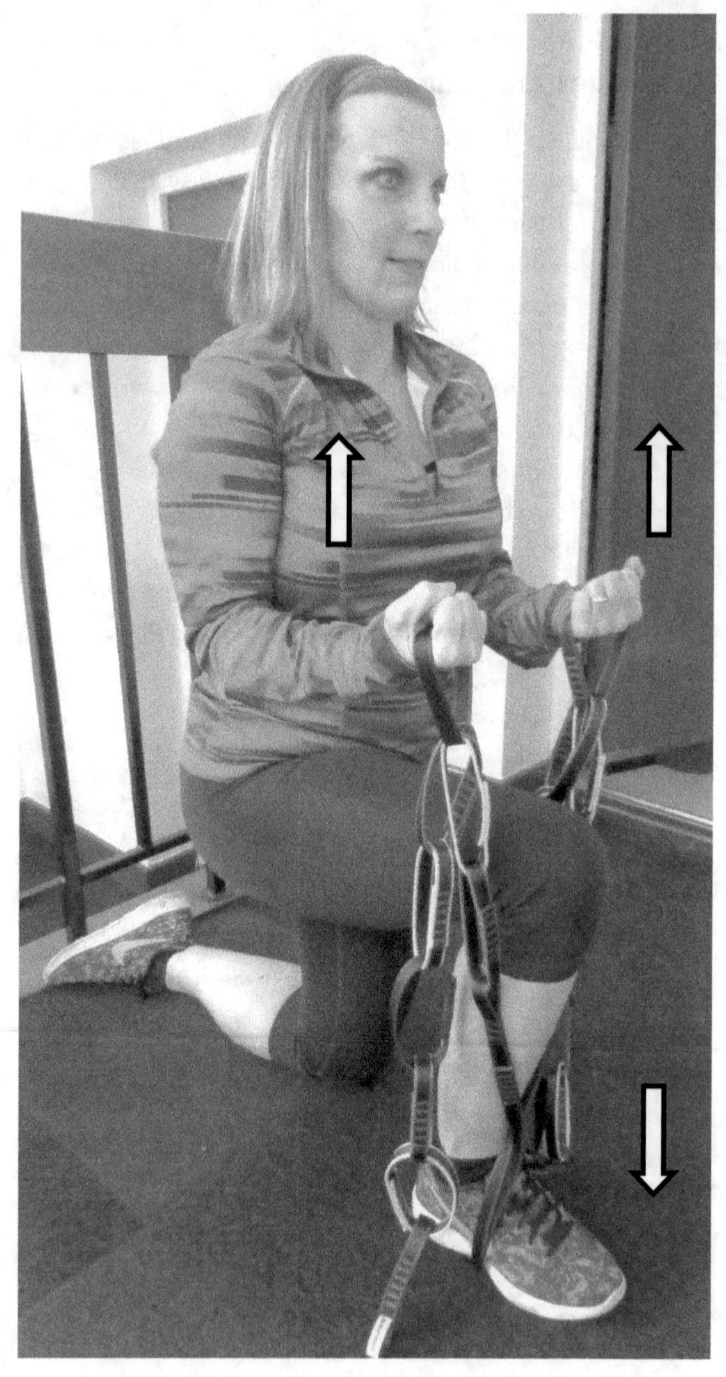

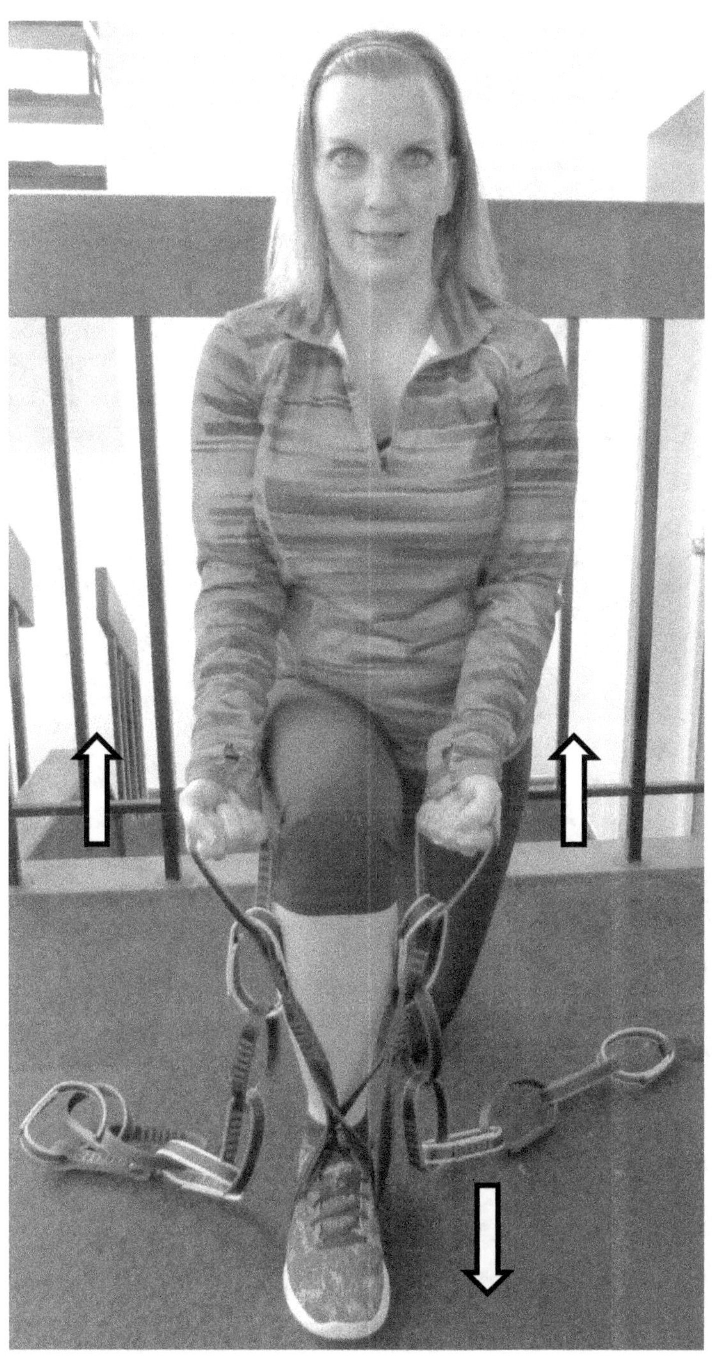

Variation – Single Arm Kneeling Curl

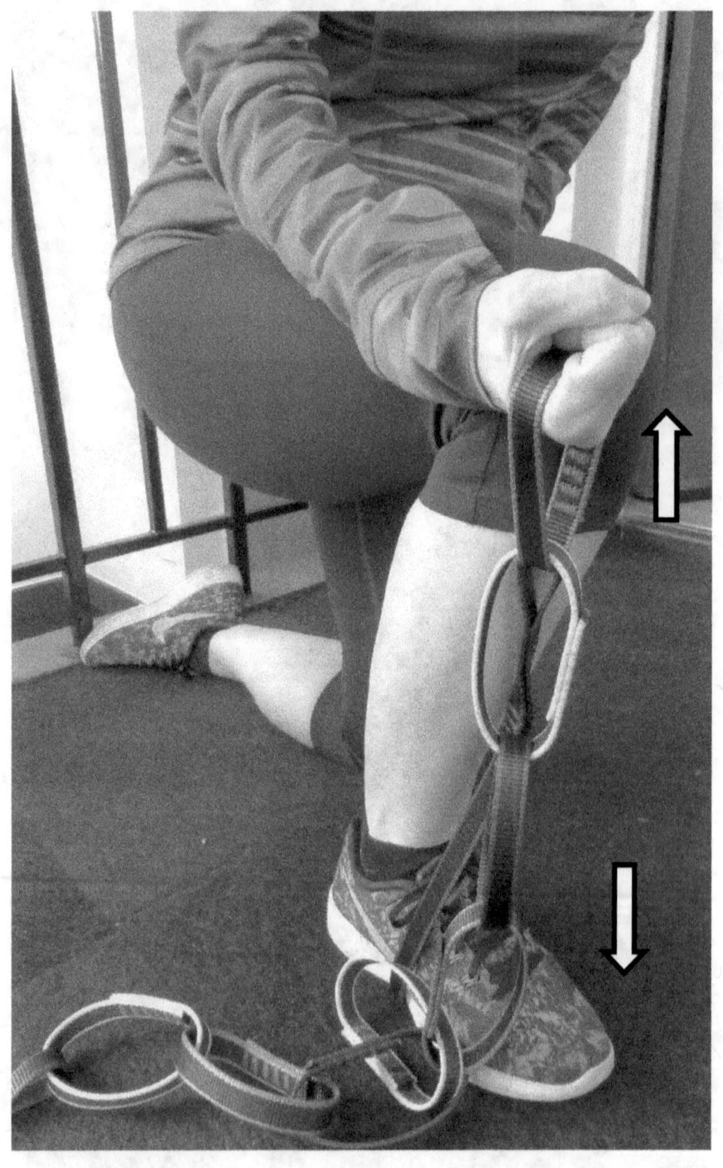

Section 2 Biceps:
Standing Leg-Resisted Curl (Both Arms)

Stand upright, and if needed, lean against a wall or any other safe, solid object to aid your stability. Place the foot loop of each daisy chain around one raised foot. Grip with palms facing upwards, the same coloured loop of each daisy chain on each side of the leg. For general exercise, choose a loop that allows you to perform an exercise at approximately the midpoint. In this position, keep your elbows back and at the side of your body as you attempt to perform a biceps curl with the weight and muscles of your leg, providing immovable resistance. When you perform an isometric exercise, never hold your breath. Always breathe deeply and naturally, which will be about 10 full breaths at a rate of about 1 second per breath. Perform each exercise

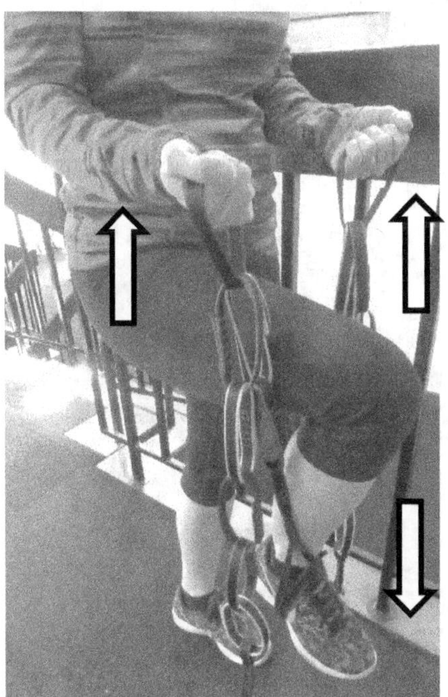

for no less than 7 seconds and no longer than 10.

Note: If you are using a single daisy chain, remember to exercise both arms/sides. Advanced users can perform the exercise using different loop positions to exercise the biceps muscles at different angles on the ROM, or Range of Motion.

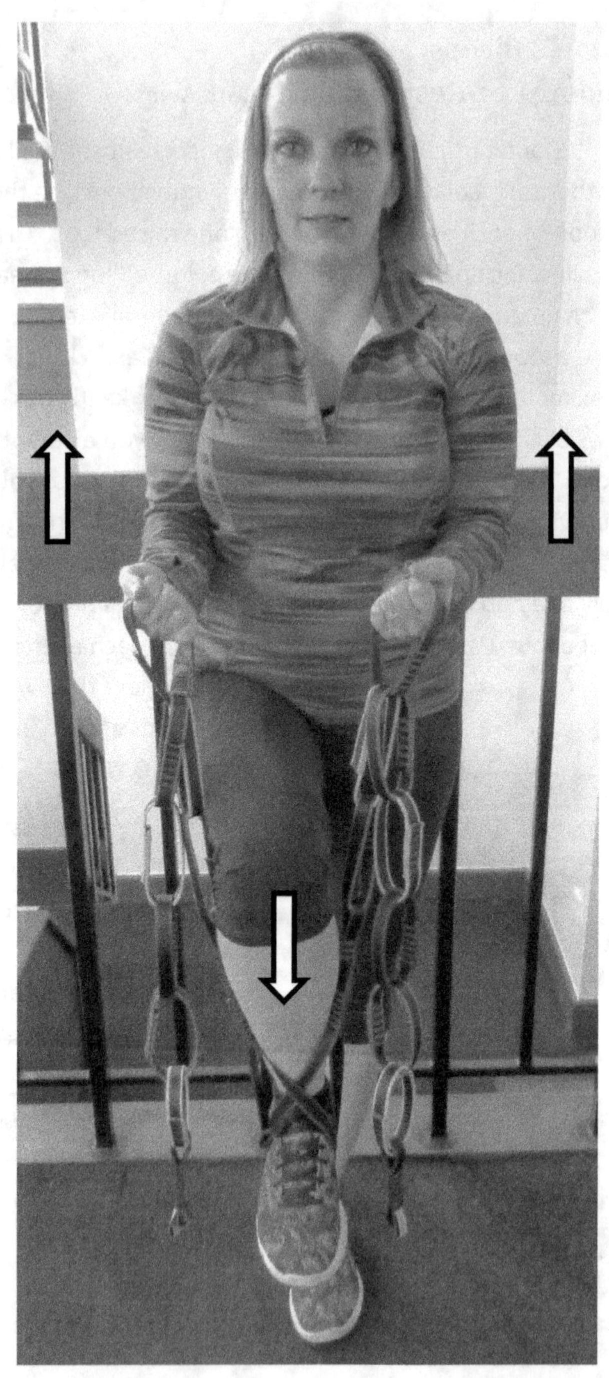

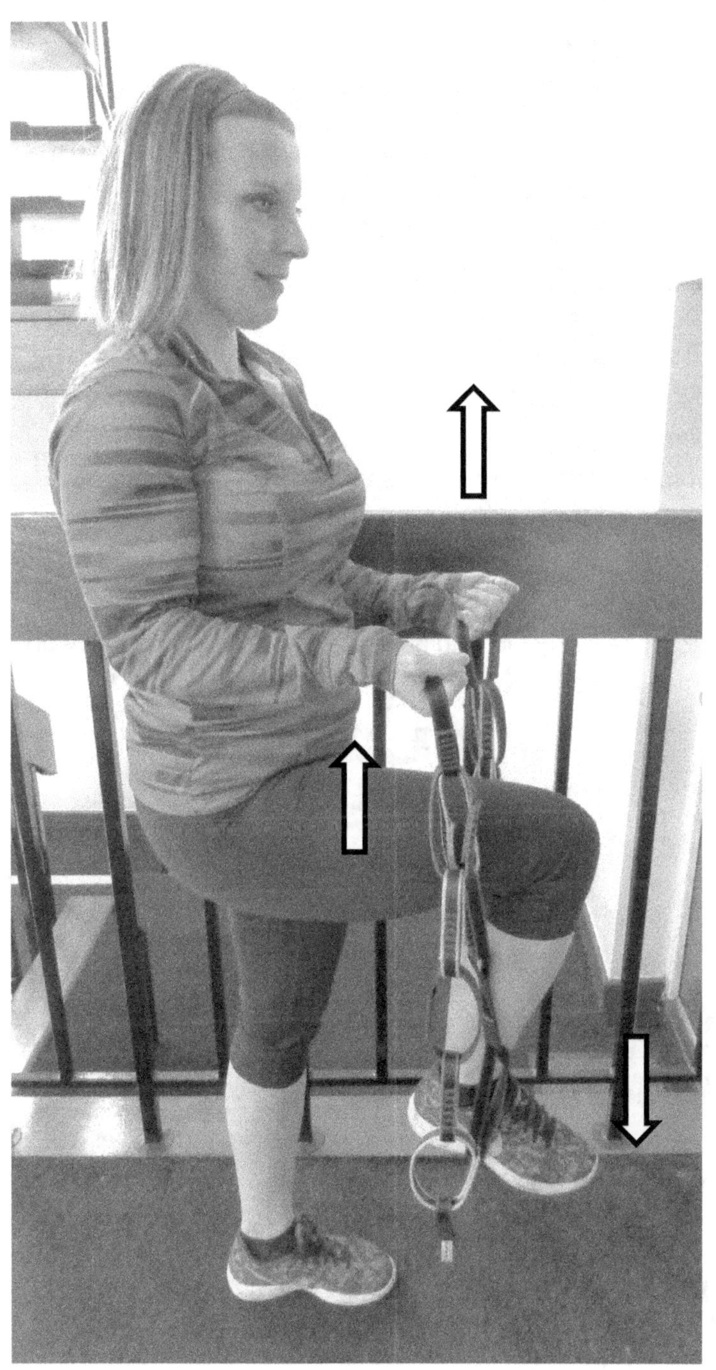

Section 2 Biceps:
Standing Biceps Curl (Both Arms)

Stand upright and place the foot loop of each daisy chain around each foot. Grip with palms facing upwards, the same coloured loop of each daisy chain on each side of the leg. For general exercise, choose a loop that allows you to perform an exercise at approximately the midpoint. In this position, keep your elbows back and at the side of your body as you attempt to perform a biceps curl with the weight and muscles of your legs and feet, providing immovable resistance. When you perform an isometric exercise, never hold your breath. Always breathe deeply and naturally, which will be about 10 full breaths at a rate of about 1 second per breath. Perform each exercise for no less than 7 seconds and no longer than 10. Note: If you are using a single daisy chain, do not forget to exercise both arms/sides. Also, advanced users can perform the exercise using different loop positions to exercise the biceps muscles at different angles on the ROM or Range of Motion.

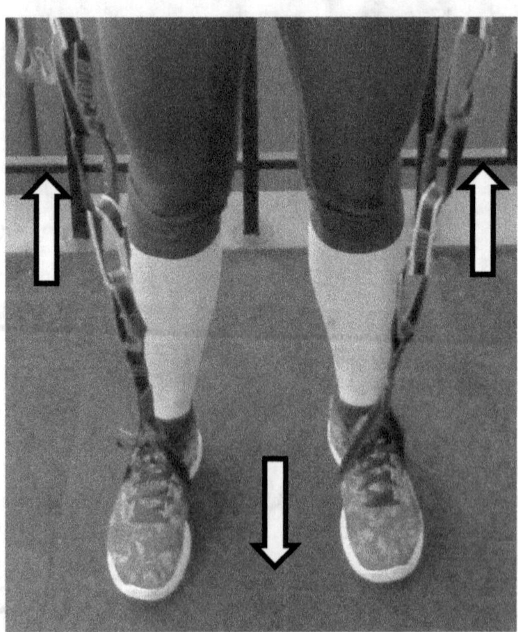

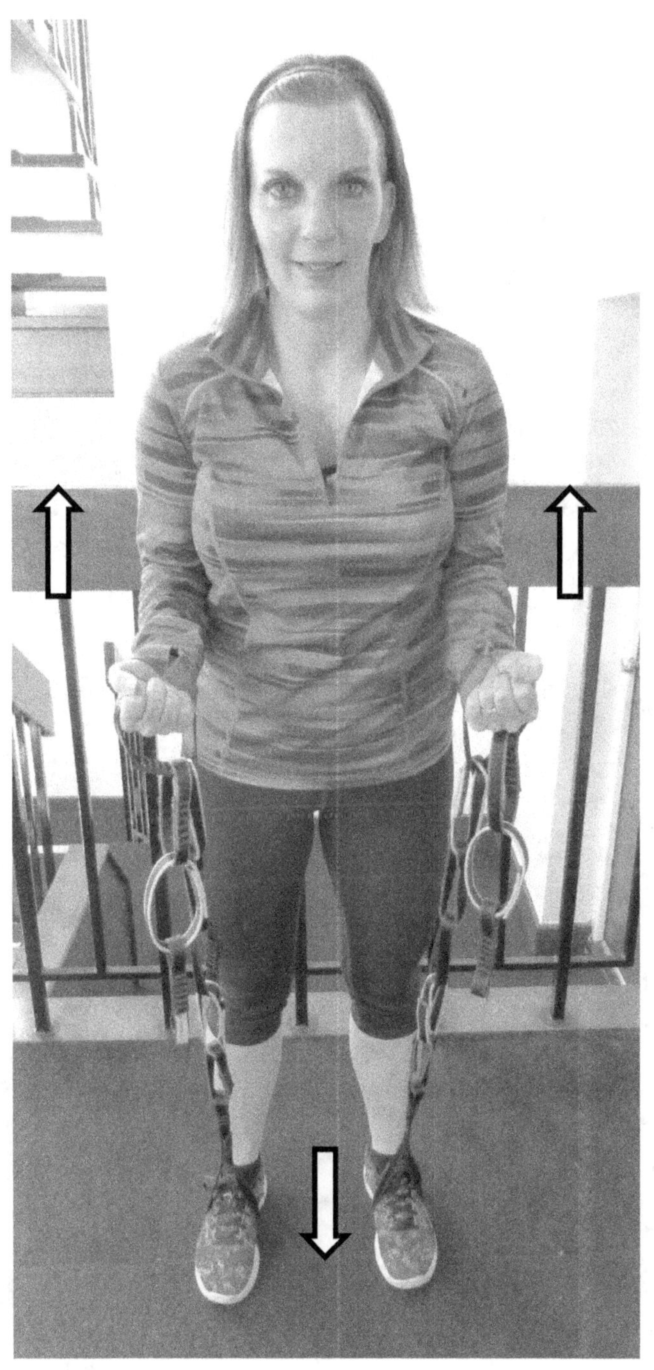

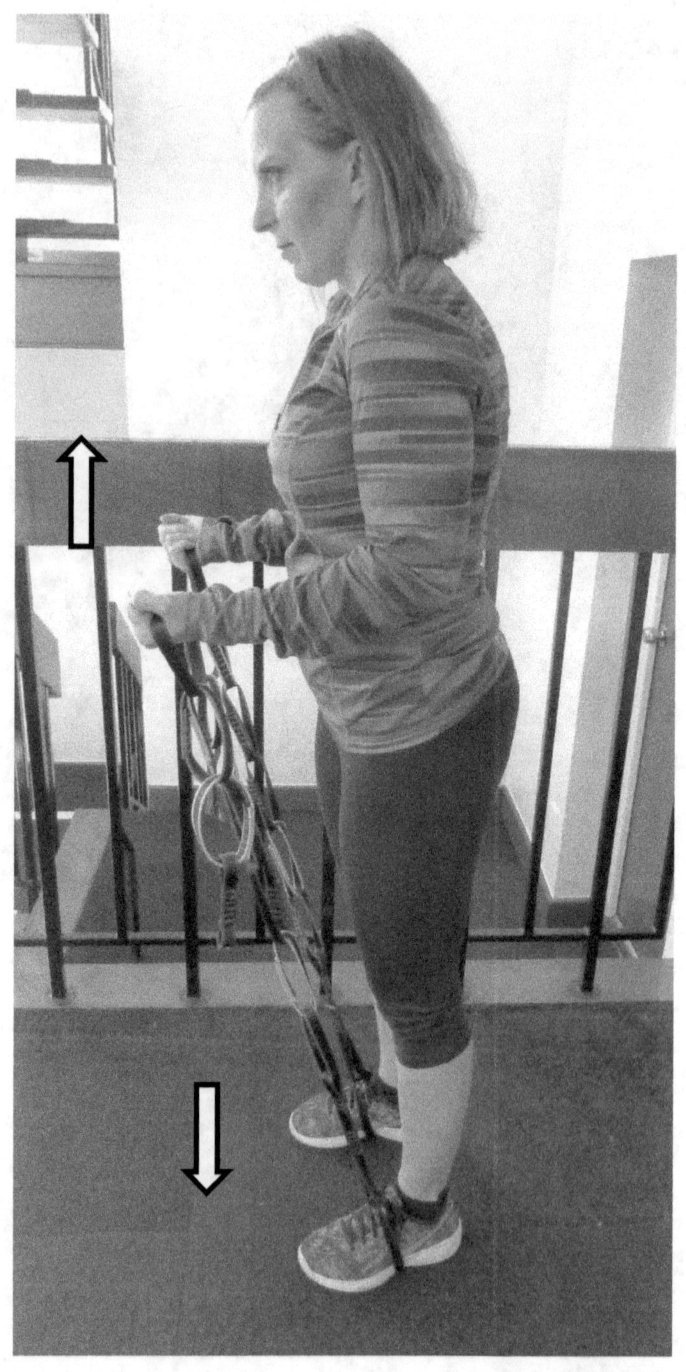

105

Section 2 Biceps Variations: Advanced Multi-Angle Standing Biceps Curl (Both Arms)

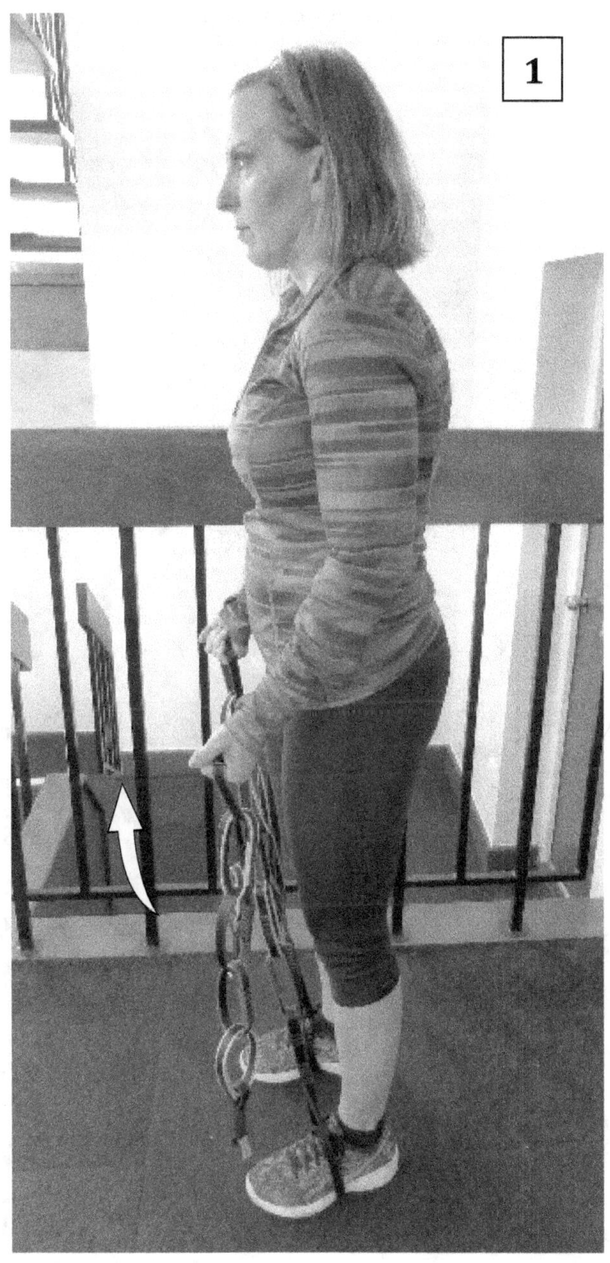

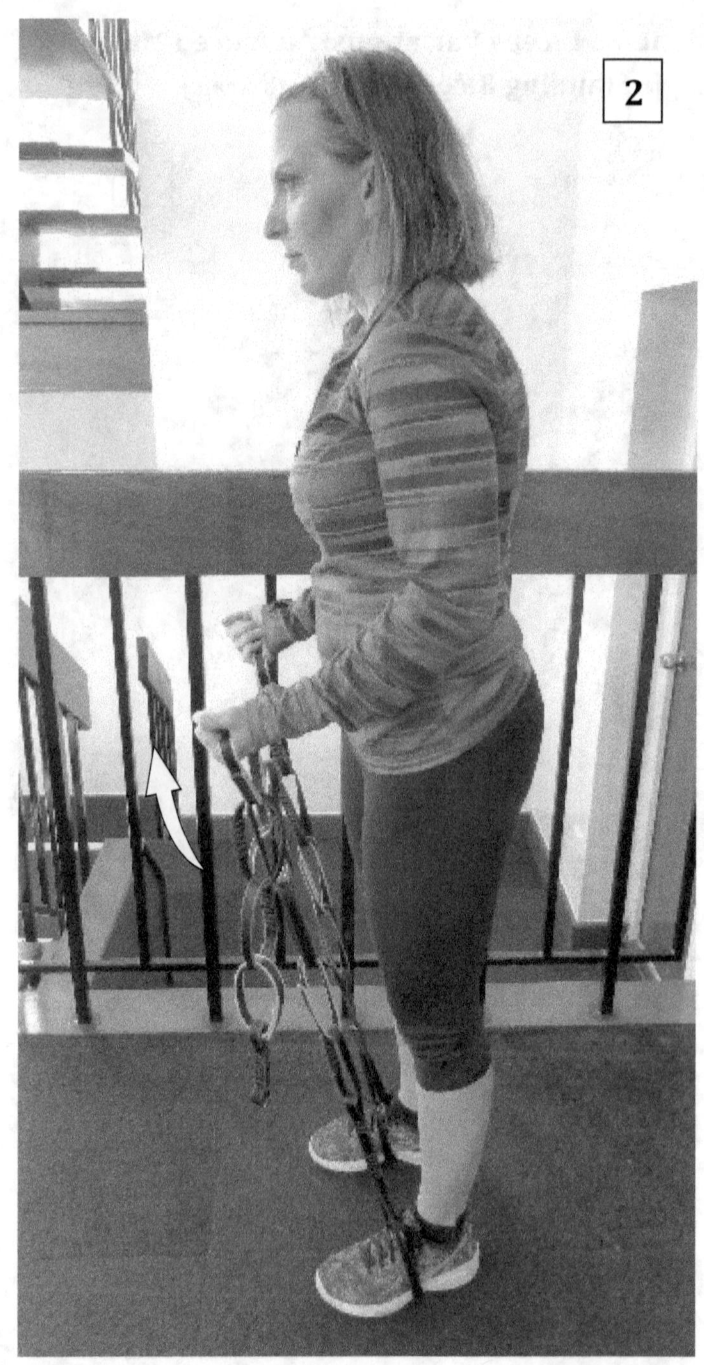

2

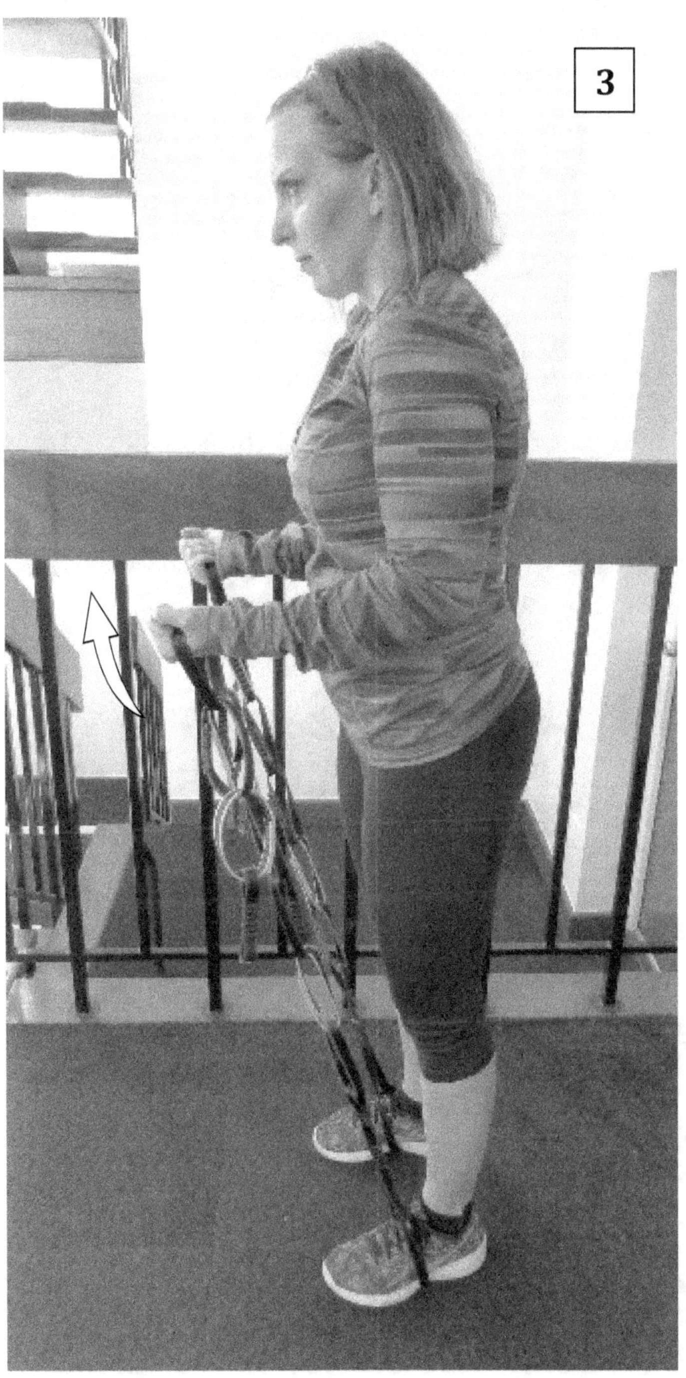

3

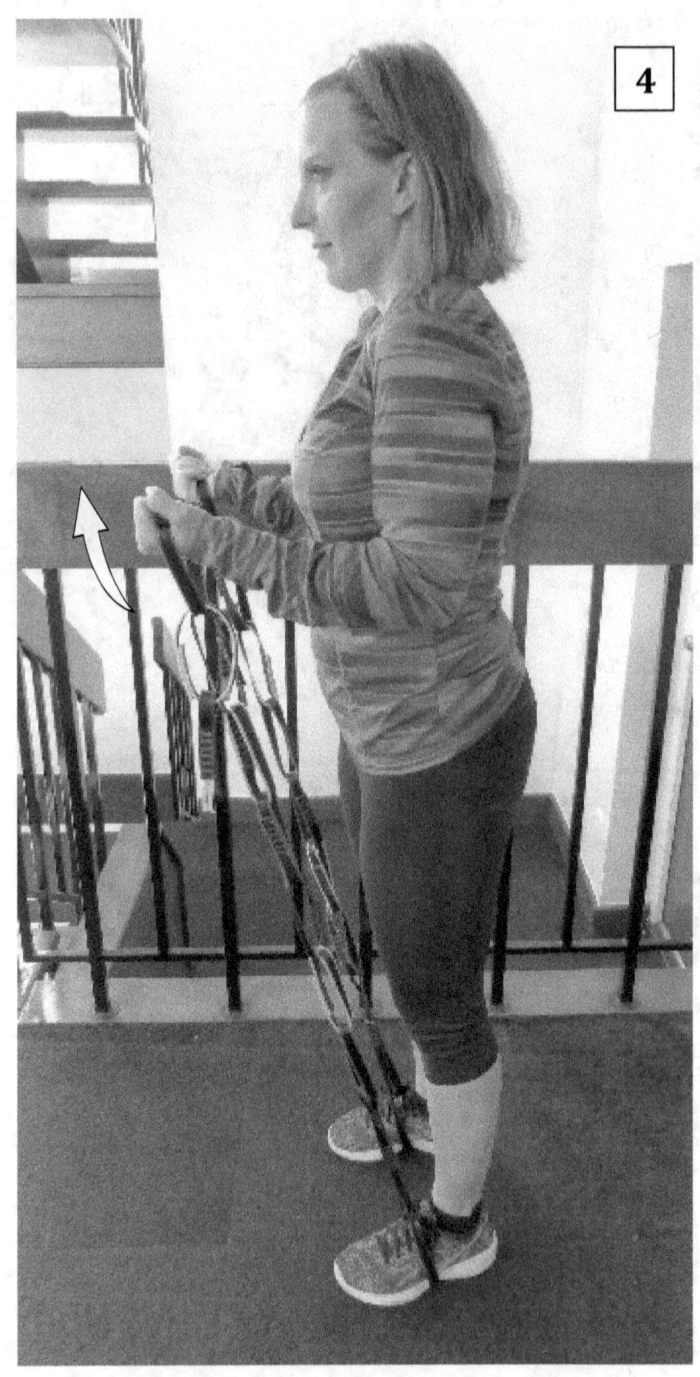

4

Sections 2 & 3 Simultaneous Exercise

Biceps and Triceps Dual Self-Resistance
(Left and Right Side)

The biceps and triceps dual resistance technique exercises the biceps muscles on one arm while simultaneously exercising the triceps muscles on the other arm. One hand grips a loop of the daisy chain with the palm facing downwards, while the other hand grips the same loop with the palm facing upwards.

Both arms and elbows must always remain close to the body, with the elbows bent enough to allow the muscles to be exercised properly. An advanced variant would be to perform the same exercises in each of three consecutive daisy chain loops. This will give a lower, mid, and upper position on the ROM or Range of Motion.

When you perform an isometric exercise, never hold your breath. Always breathe deeply and naturally, which will be about 10 full breaths at a rate of about 1 second per breath. Perform each exercise for no less than 7 seconds and no longer than 10. Also, remember to change from palms up to palms down on each hand/side to exercise the biceps and triceps of both arms in the same way.

Note: Some people prefer to perform this exercise with the hands positioned roughly along the midline at the front of the body or with alternate hands/arms at opposing sides of the body. Both methods are fine, but finding a position that works best for you is more important. Never allow your wrists to bend backwards during any exercise, as this reduces the level of force that can be applied.

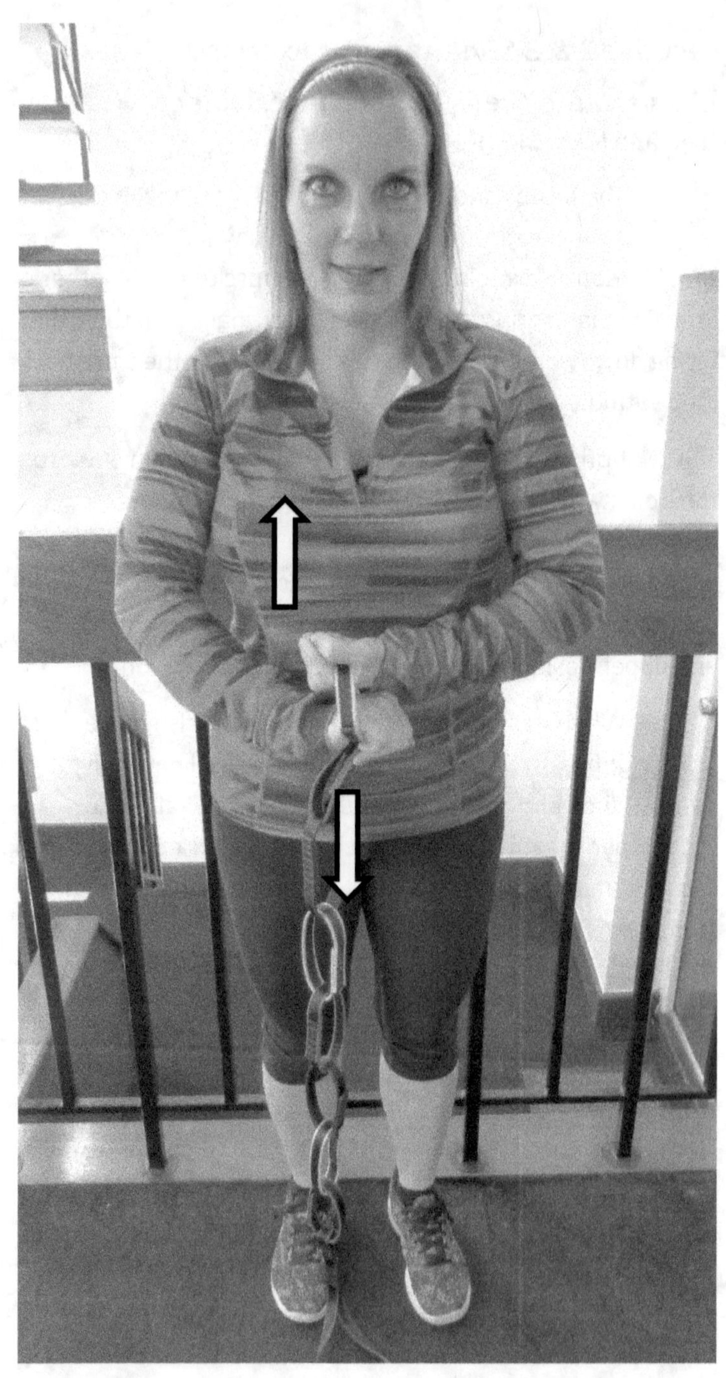

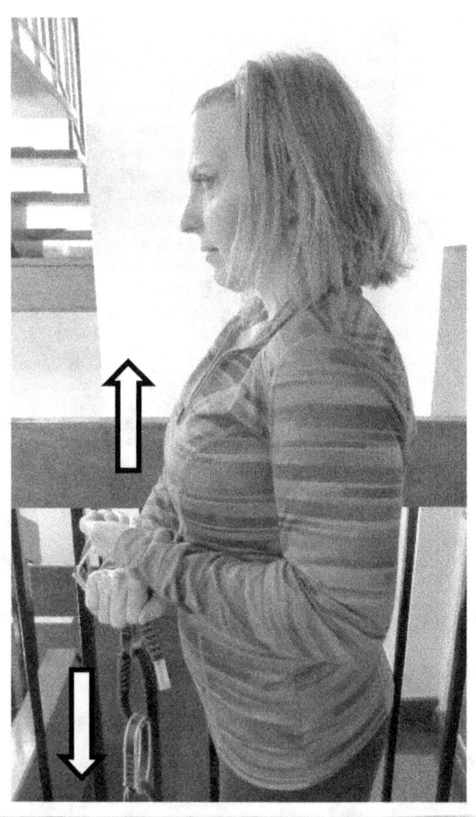

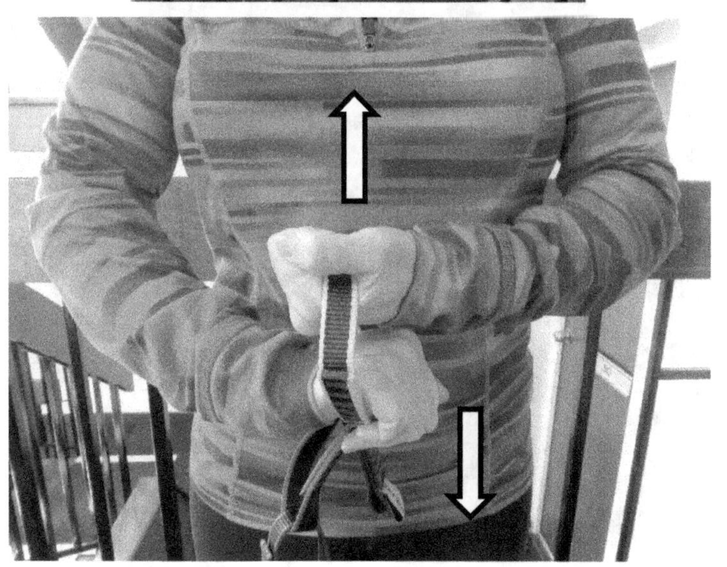

Advanced Variations From Using the Single Loop to Other Wider-Spaced Loops

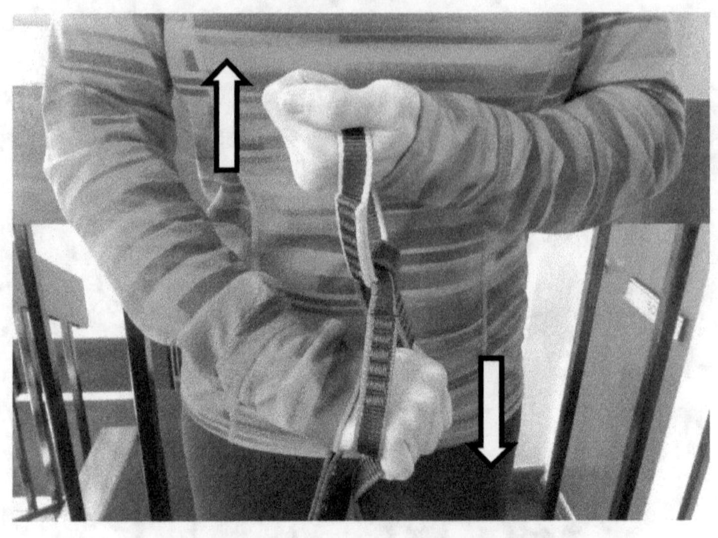

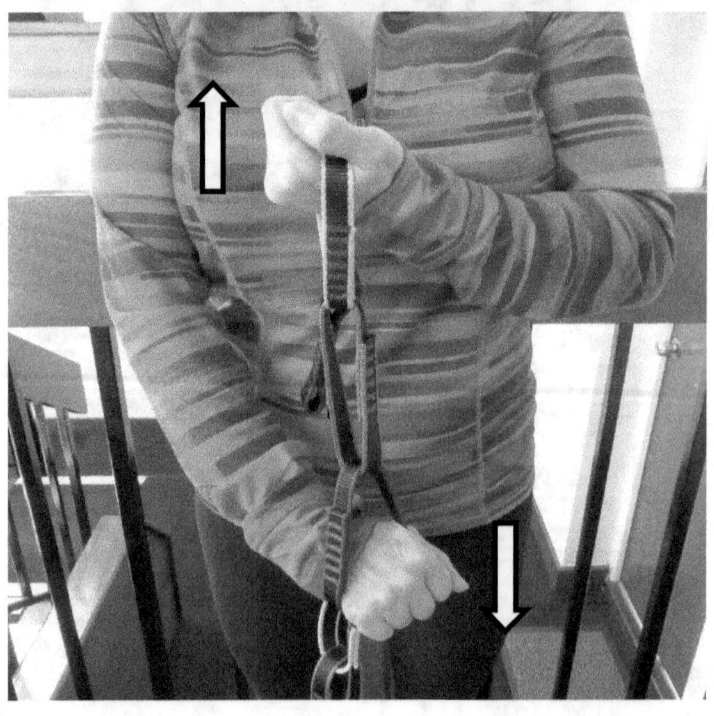

Section 3 Triceps:

Forward Triceps Press with Both Arms

Hold a loop in each hand and position the daisy chain securely across the upper-mid part of your back so it will not slip. Take a loop position that allows you to raise your upper arms so they are as forward as possible. With both elbows raised and pointing forward, be sure to keep them close together to focus the exercise on your triceps muscles. If they are allowed to spread apart sideways, then this focus will be lost. In this position, perform a triceps forward press with both arms. This will be a similar action to that of a traditional lying triceps press/extension with a barbell. Both elbows must remain bent enough to exercise the muscles properly.

An advanced variant would be to perform the same exercises in each of three consecutive daisy chain loops. This will give a lower, mid, and upper position on the ROM or Range of Motion. This exercise works equally well when performing a triceps press with both arms and a single arm. If you are performing the single-arm variant, be sure to adjust the grip position of your securing hand/arm and exercise both arms.

When you perform an isometric exercise, never hold your breath. Always breathe deeply and naturally, which will be about 10 full breaths at a rate of about 1 second per breath. Perform each exercise for no less than 7 seconds and no longer than 10.

Note: Never allow your wrists to bend backwards during any exercise, as this reduces the level of force that can be applied.

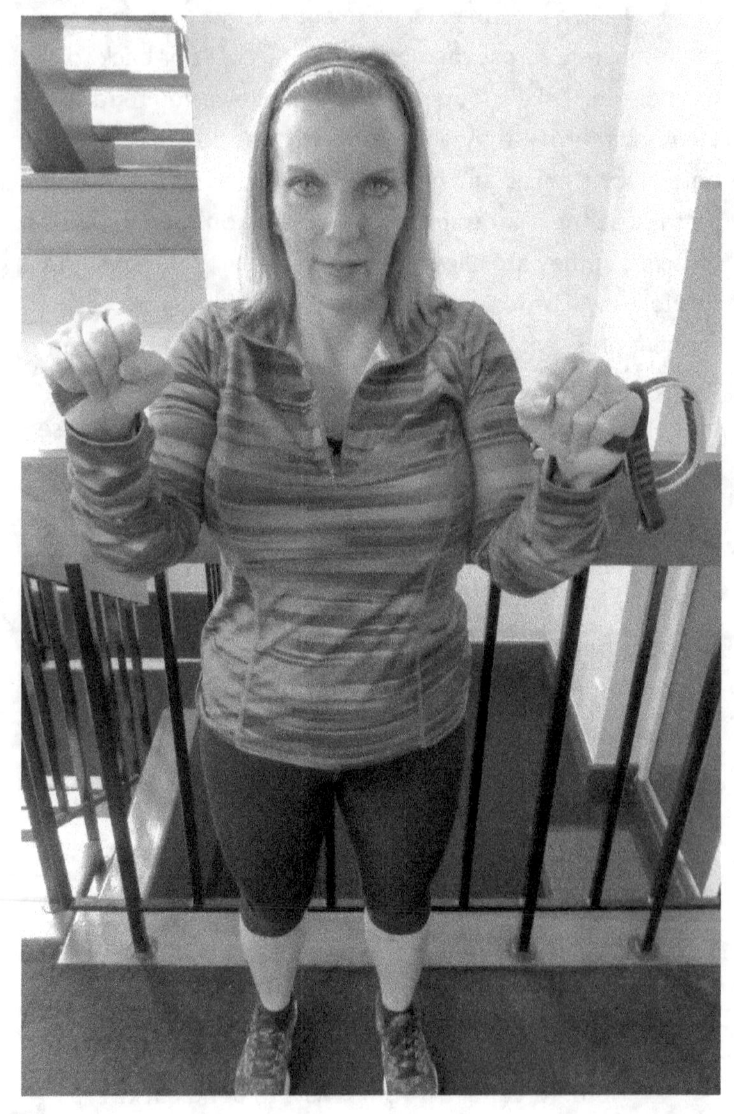

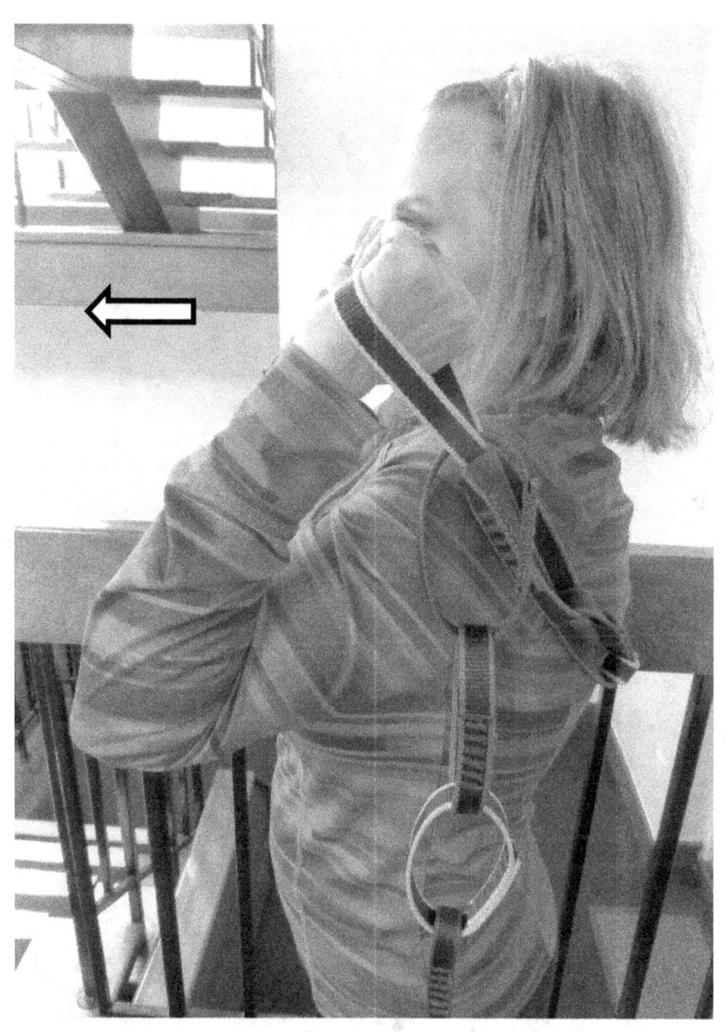

Advanced Variations Would Use Other Loops, Allowing the Triceps to be Exercised at Different Points on the Arm's ROM – Range of Motion

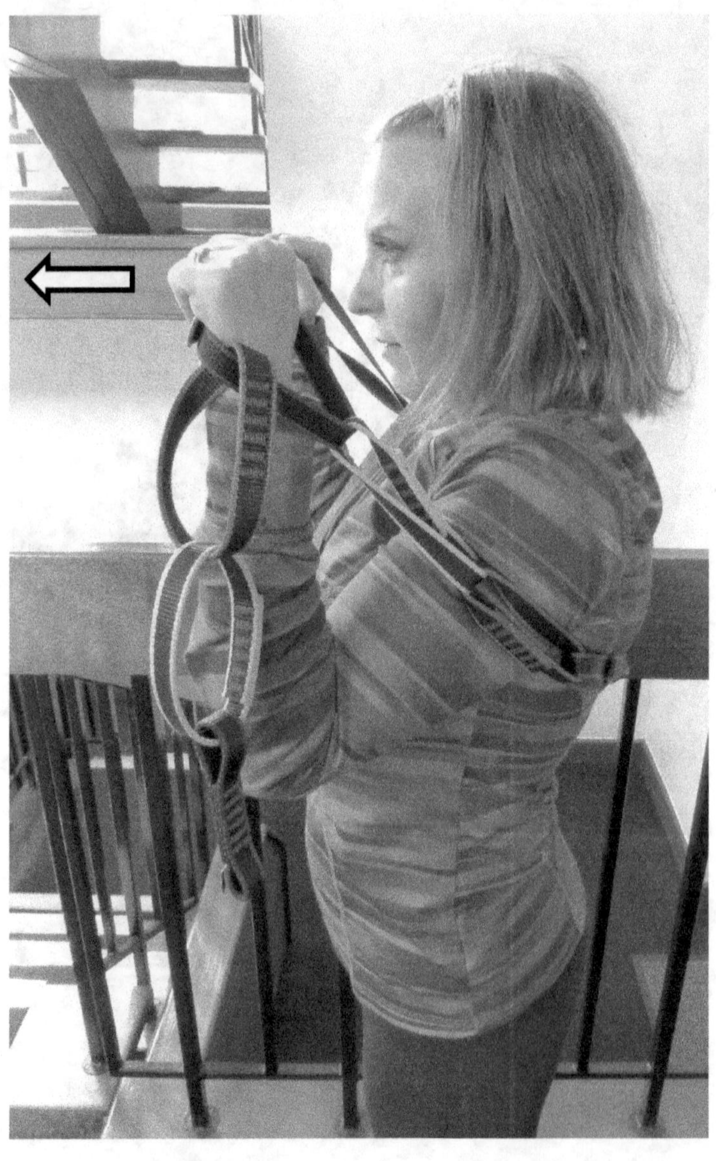

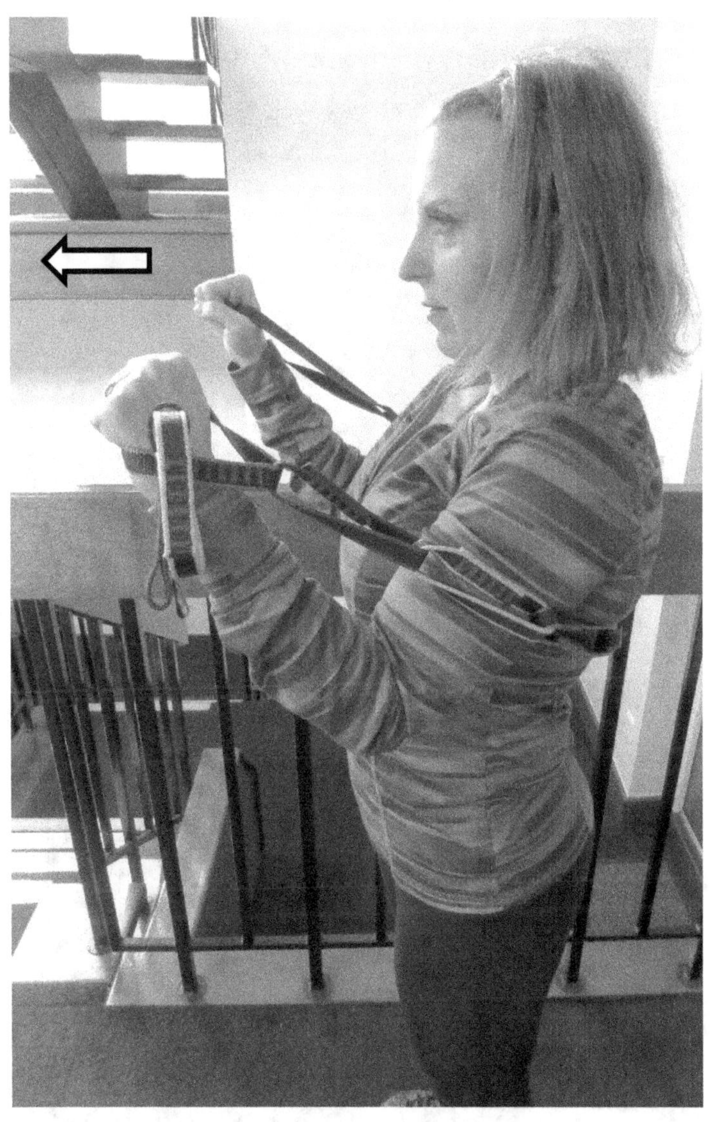

118

**Single Arm Forward Triceps Press
(Exercise Both Arms)**

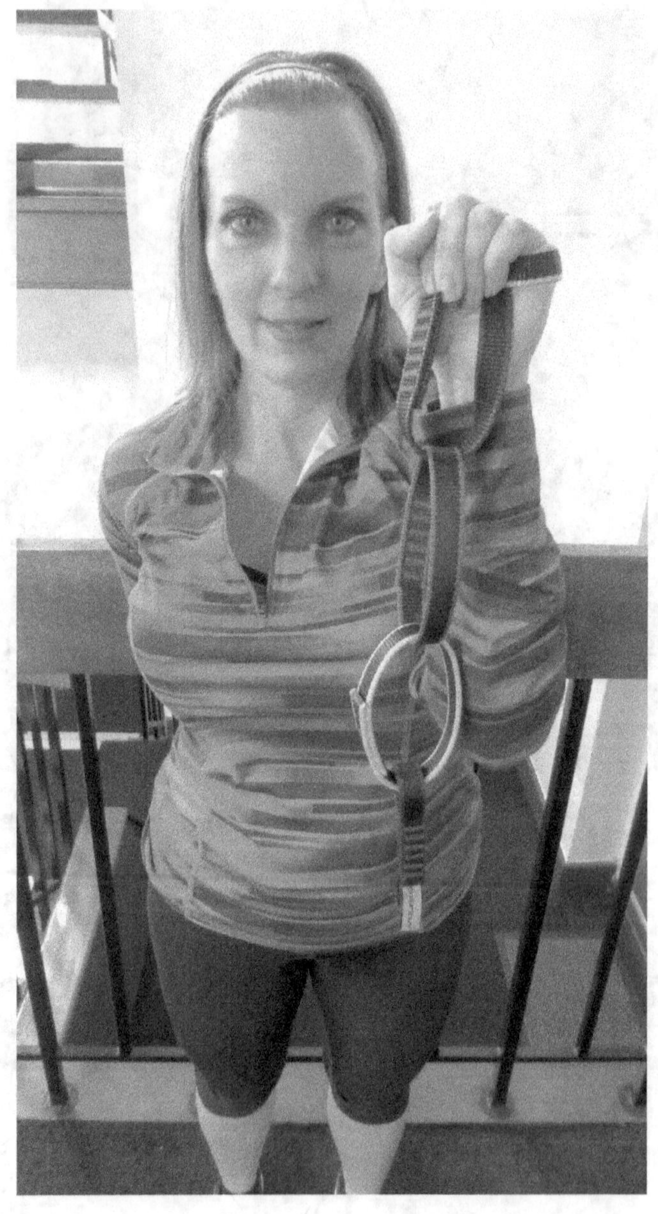

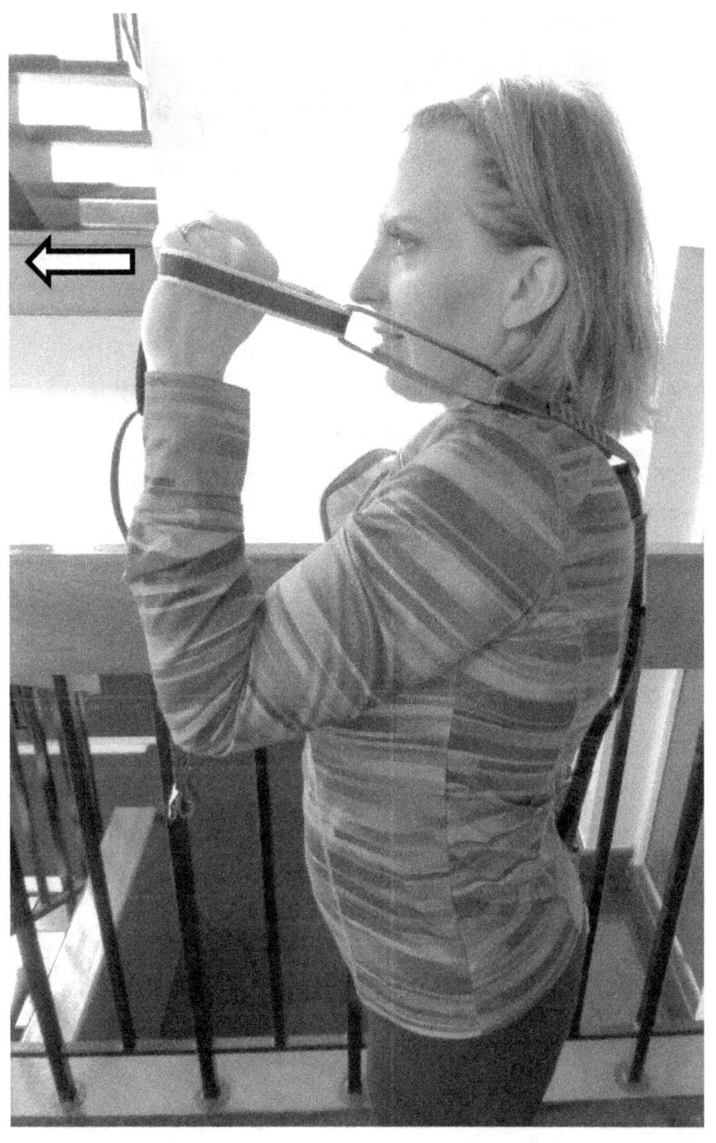

Section 3 Triceps:

Overhead Triceps Press Single Arm
(Left and Right Side)

Hold a daisy chain loop in one hand with your arm above your head so that your upper arm is as close to vertical as possible.

Your elbow should be pointing directly upward as far as possible. Grip the lower part of the daisy chain with your other hand around the mid or lower back.

The hand that is held above your head can then engage the triceps muscles to perform an isometric extension exercise. Exercising with your hand at approximately the mid-point position will exercise the triceps in a general way.

However, advanced users can perform the same exercise with different daisy chain loops to exercise the triceps muscles at different points on the arm's ROM, or Range of Motion.

When you perform an isometric exercise, never hold your breath. Always breathe deeply and naturally, which will be about 10 full breaths at a rate of about 1 second per breath. Perform each exercise for no less than 7 seconds and no longer than 10.

Note: Never allow your wrists to bend backwards during any exercise, as this reduces the level of force that can be applied.

Also, do not forget to exercise the other arm in the same way to maintain balanced development.

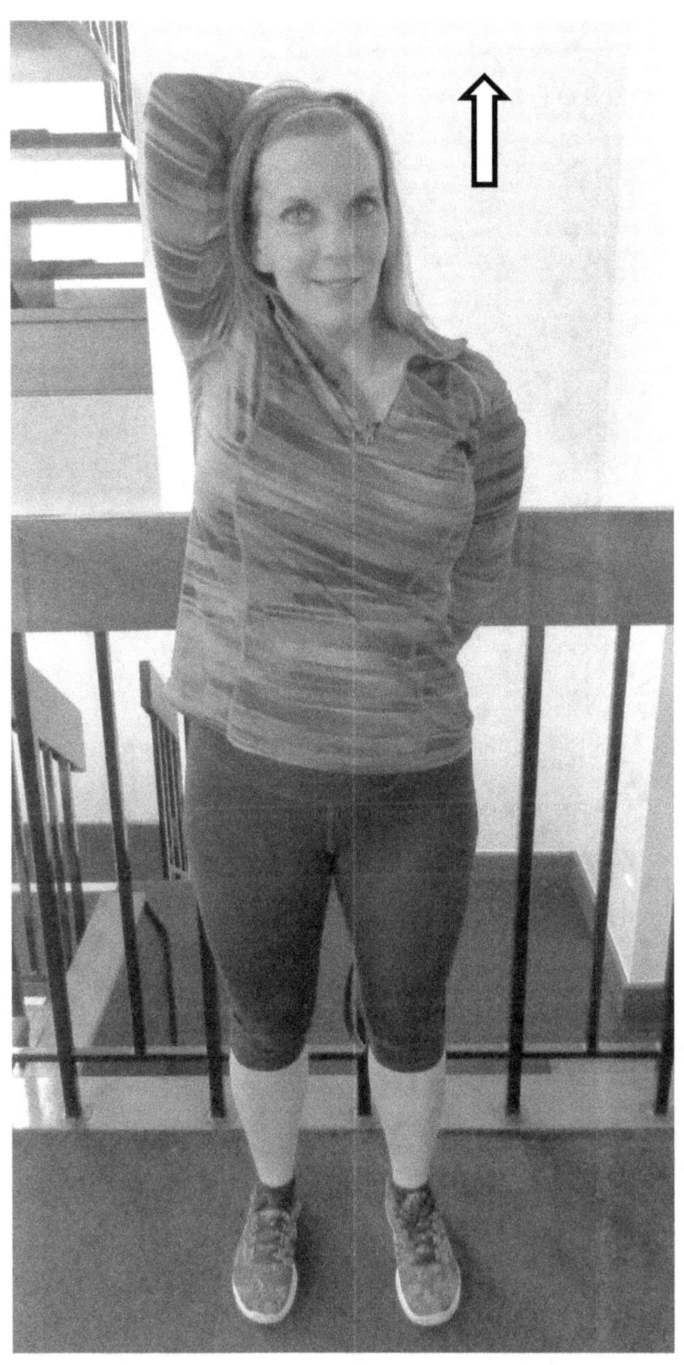

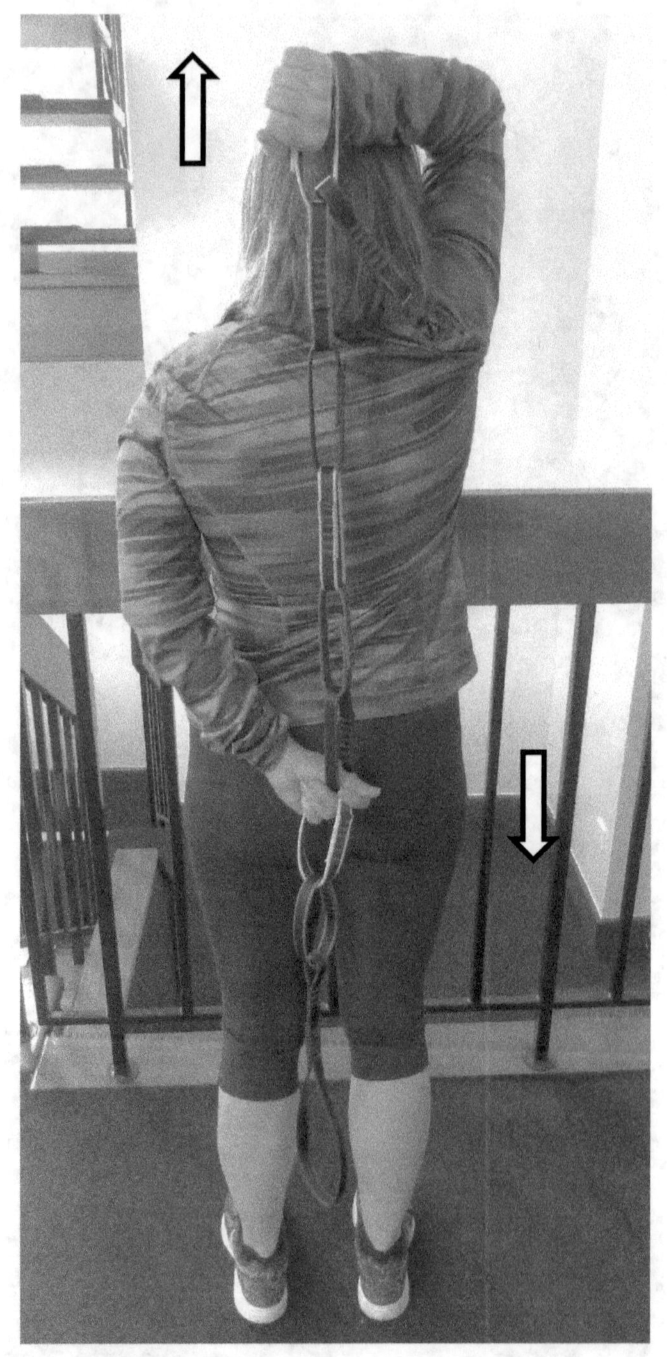

123

Advanced Variations Would Use Other Loops, Allowing the Triceps to be Exercised at Different Points on the Arm's ROM – Range of Motion

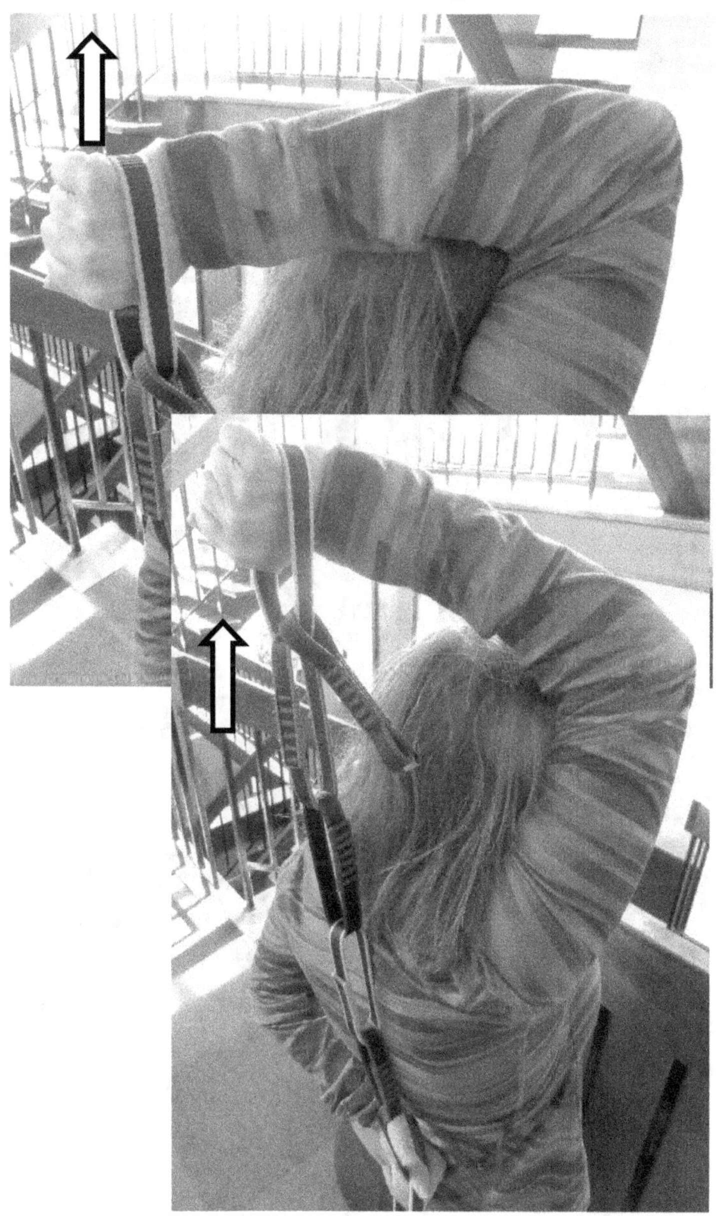

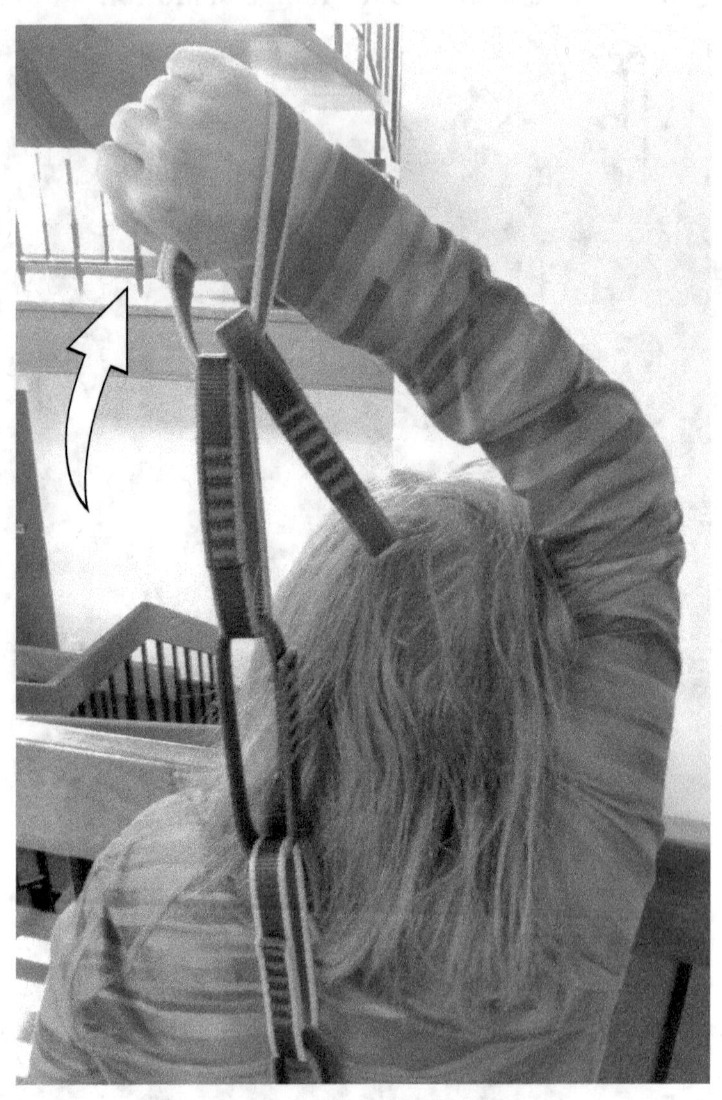

125

Section 3 Triceps:

Triceps Forward Press Down Single Arm
(Left and Right Side)

Hold a daisy chain loop in one hand, palm facing down, and with the rest of the daisy chain over your shoulder. Grip the other end of the daisy chain with your other hand at either the mid-point or the lower back. Keep your forward arm close to the body with your elbow bent at approximately 90 degrees. Use the triceps muscles of the forward arm to press downwards to perform the isometric exercise. Your hand at approximately the mid-point position will exercise the triceps in a general way. However, advanced users can perform the same exercise with different loops of the daisy chain to exercise the triceps muscles at different points on the arm's ROM, or Range of

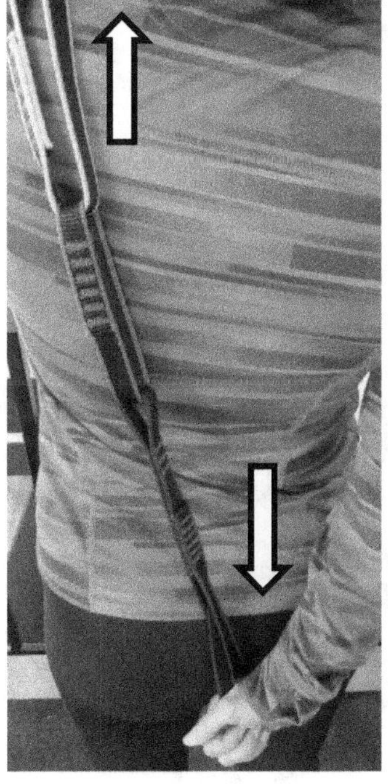

Motion. When you perform an isometric exercise, never hold your breath. Always breathe deeply and naturally, which will be about 10 full breaths at a rate of about 1 second per breath. Perform each exercise for no less than 7 seconds and no longer than 10. Note: Never allow your wrists to bend backwards during any exercise, as this reduces the level of force that can be applied. Do not forget to exercise both arms in the same way.

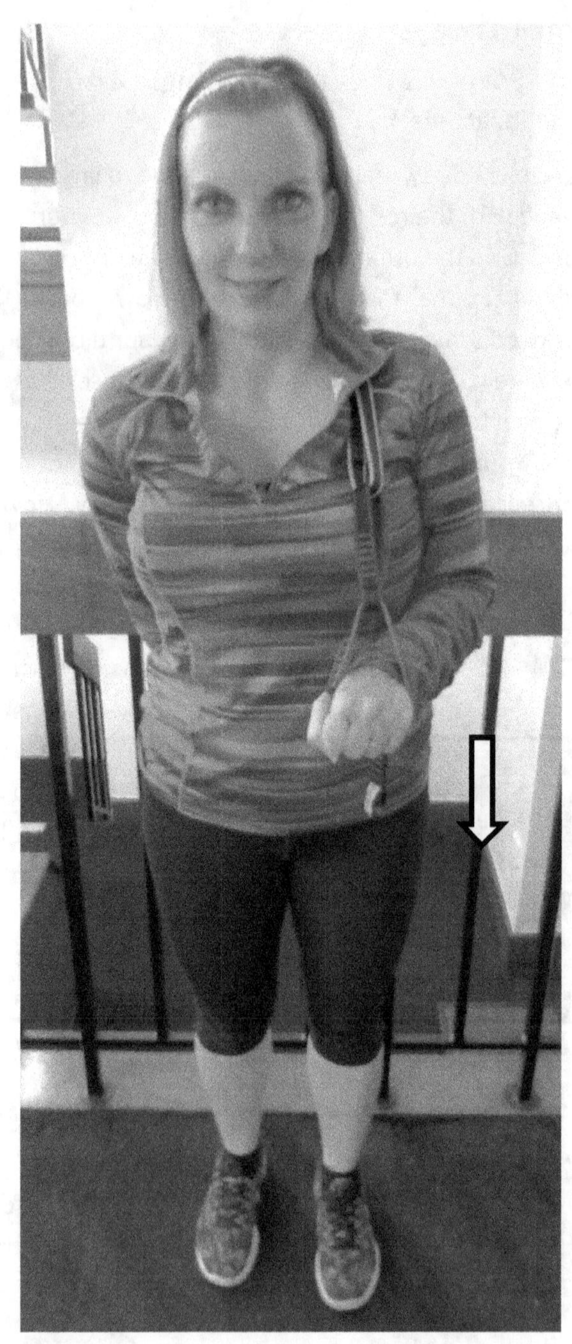

127

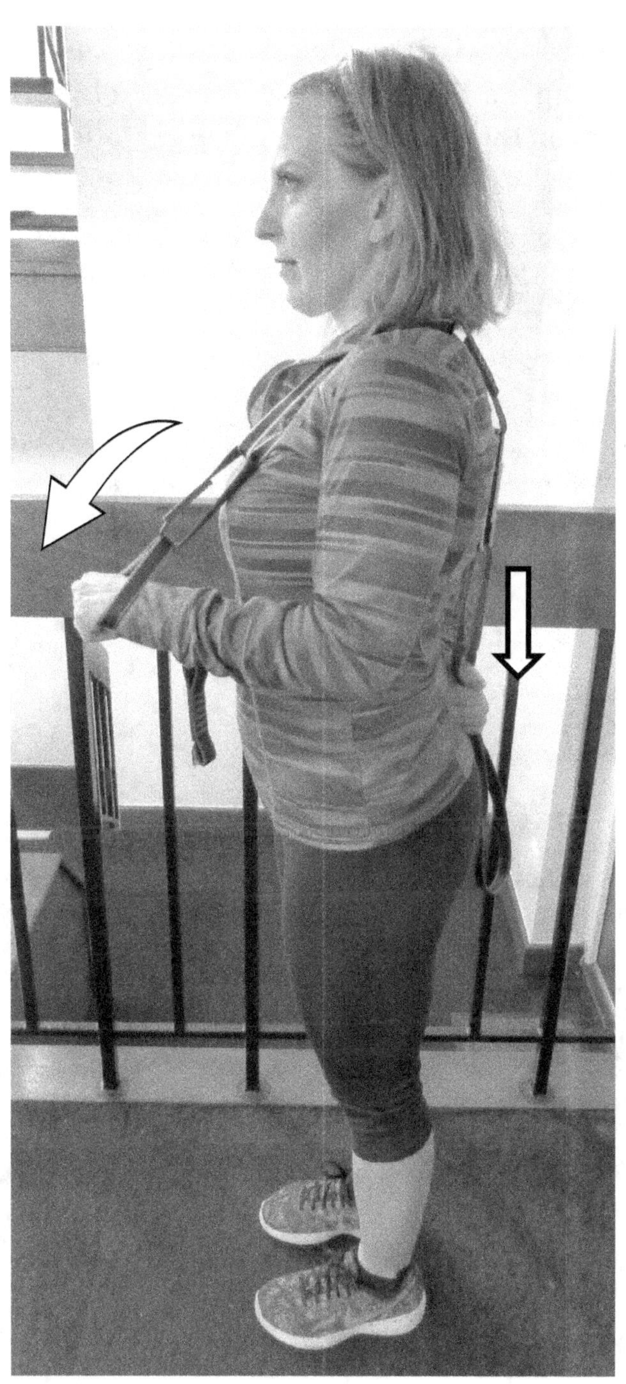

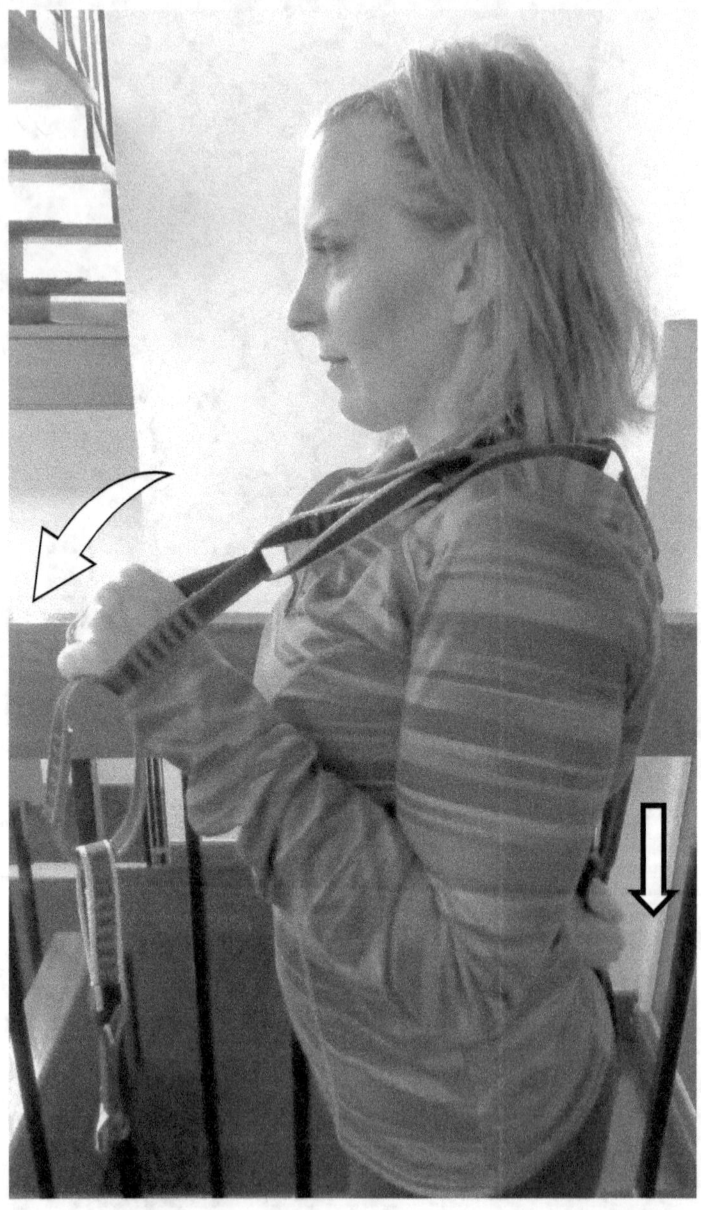

Section 3 Triceps:

Triceps Side Press Single Arm
(Left and Right Side)

Hold one end of a daisy chain at about waist level with your arm close to your body. The long end of the daisy chain should be over the shoulder of the same arm so that it loops over and across your chest.

The opposite hand can then grip an appropriately positioned loop. The hand you perform the exercise with should be held outwards and sideways, away from the body.

The upper arm should be held approximately horizontally to the floor. In this position, the exercising hand can engage the triceps muscles to perform an isometric sideways press. Your hand at approximately the mid-point position will exercise the triceps in a general way. However, advanced users can perform the same exercise with different loops of the daisy chain to exercise the triceps muscles at different points on the arm's ROM, or Range of Motion.

When you perform an isometric exercise, never hold your breath. Always breathe deeply and naturally, which will be about 10 full breaths at a rate of about 1 second per breath. Perform each exercise for no less than 7 seconds and no longer than 10.

Note: Never allow your wrists to bend backwards during any exercise, as this reduces the level of force that can be applied. Also, do not forget to exercise the other arm in the same way.

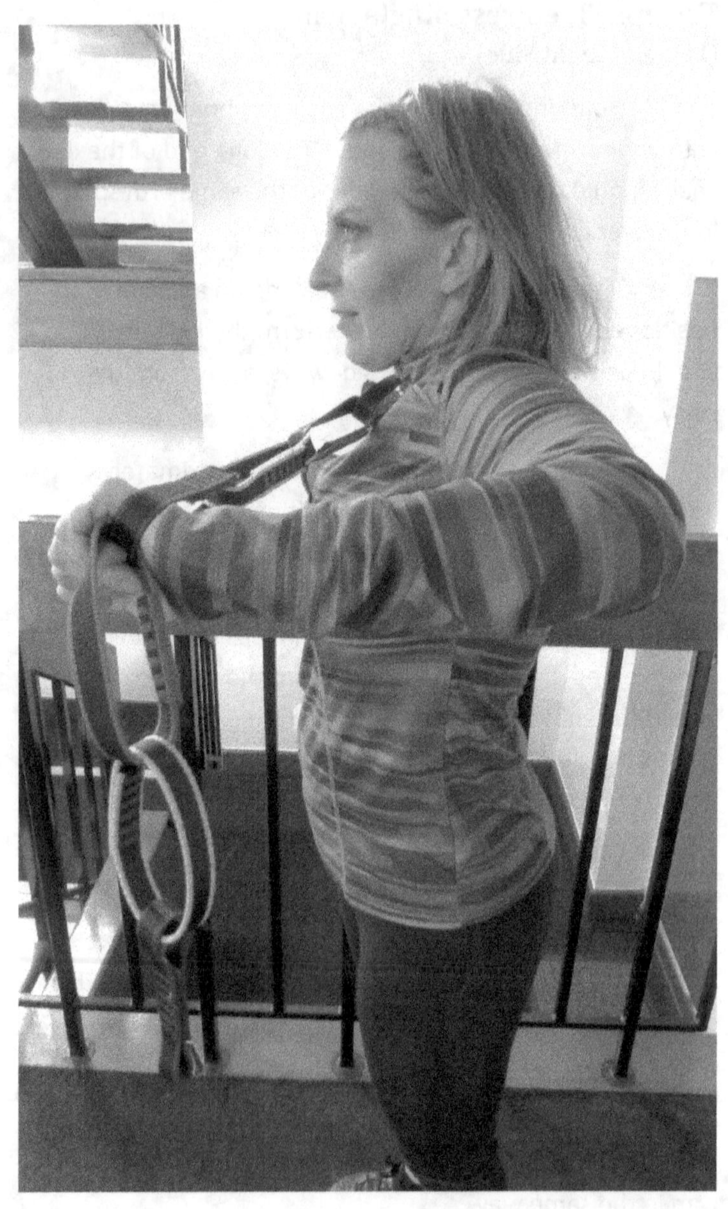

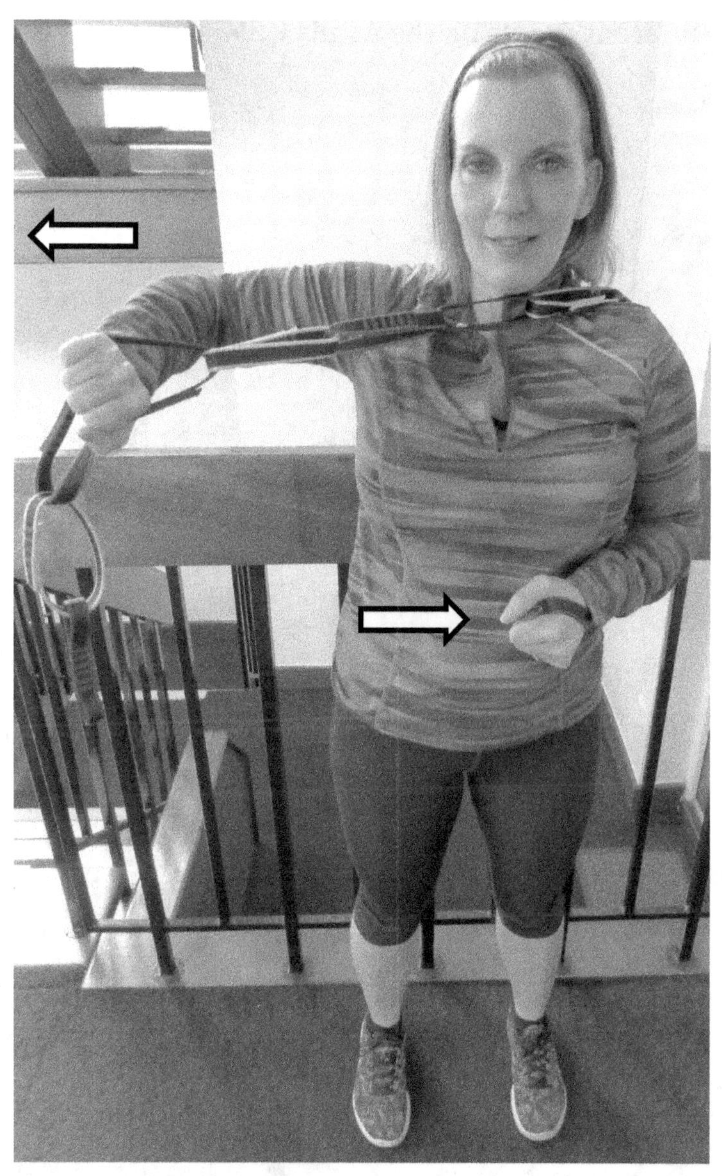

Always Exercise Both Arms and Advanced Variations Would Exercise the Triceps at Different Points on the Arm's ROM

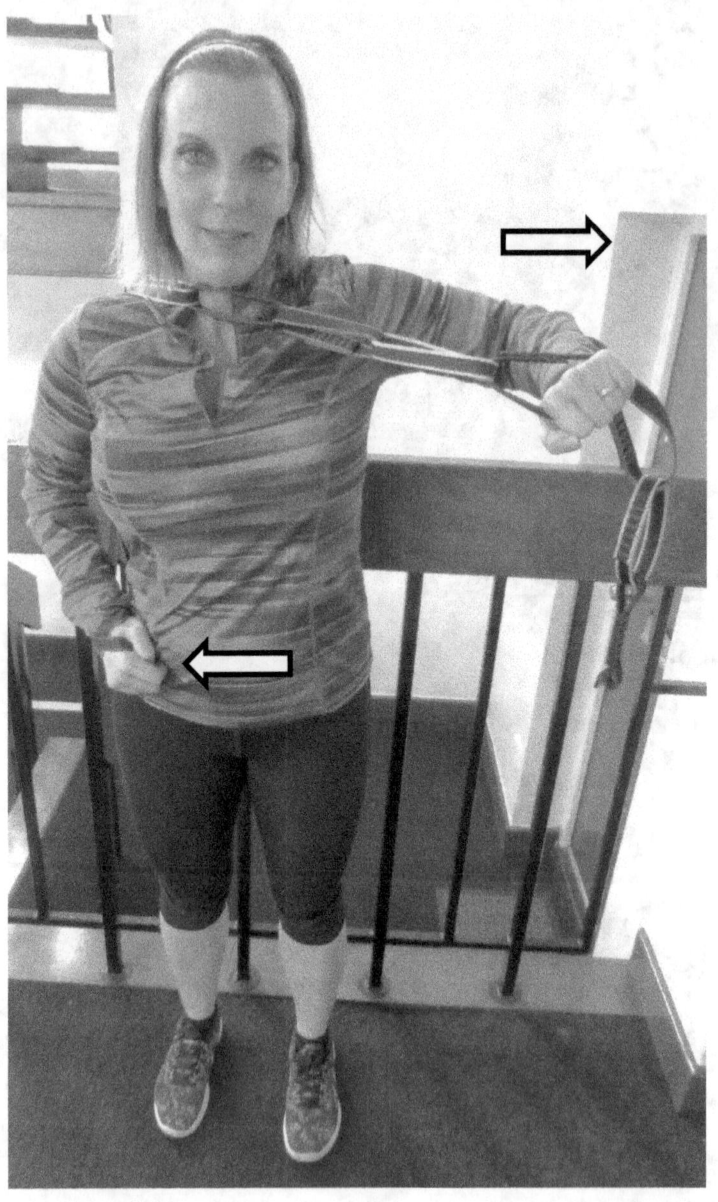

Section 4 Upper Back:

Chest-Level Upper-Back Pull-Apart

In either a seated or standing position, with your torso upright, raise your bent arms out sideways until they are roughly parallel to the floor.

Hold one loop of a daisy chain in both hands, approximately at the mid-point of the chest. In this position, apply tension to pull your hands apart. Your grip on the loop prevents this from happening as you engage the upper back, shoulder, and neck muscles.

An advanced user would perform the same exercise with wider loops. This would exercise the back at different points on the Range of Motion, or ROM.

When you perform an isometric exercise, never hold your breath. Always breathe deeply and naturally, which will be about 10 full breaths at a rate of about 1 second per breath. Perform each exercise for no less than 7 seconds and no longer than 10.

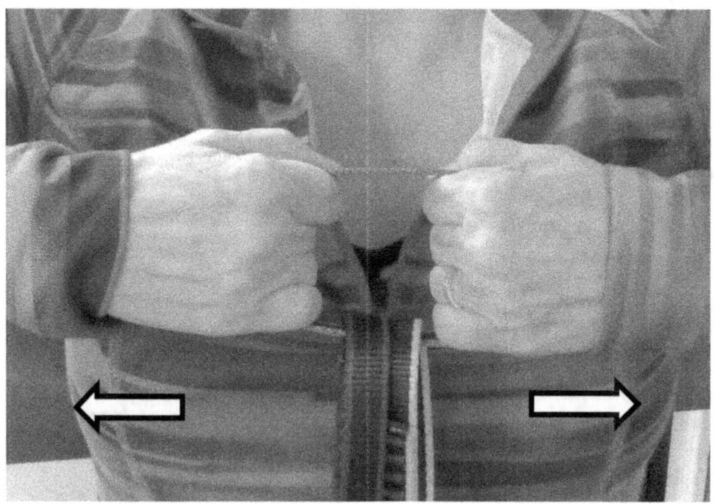

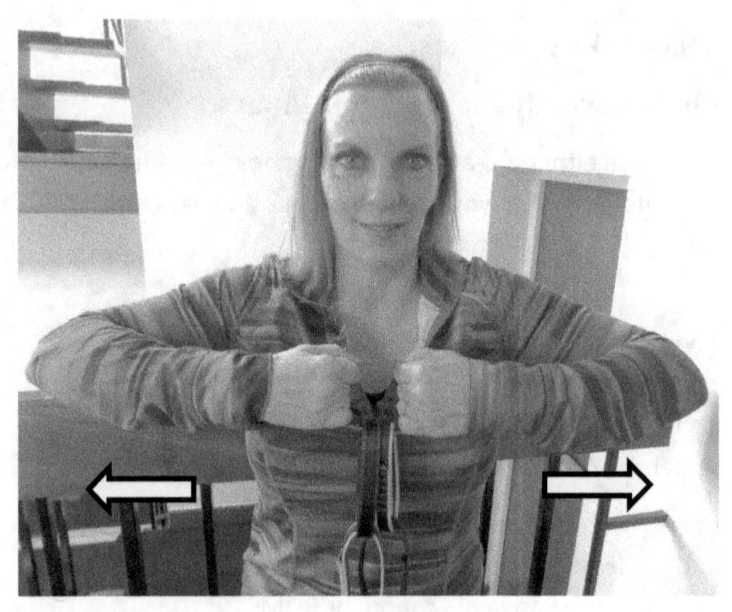

Below: Variation With Two Loops

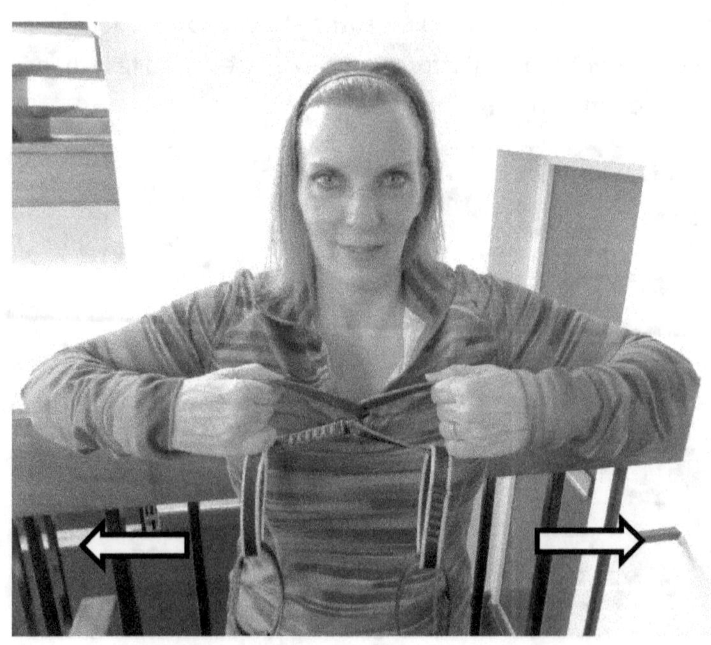

135

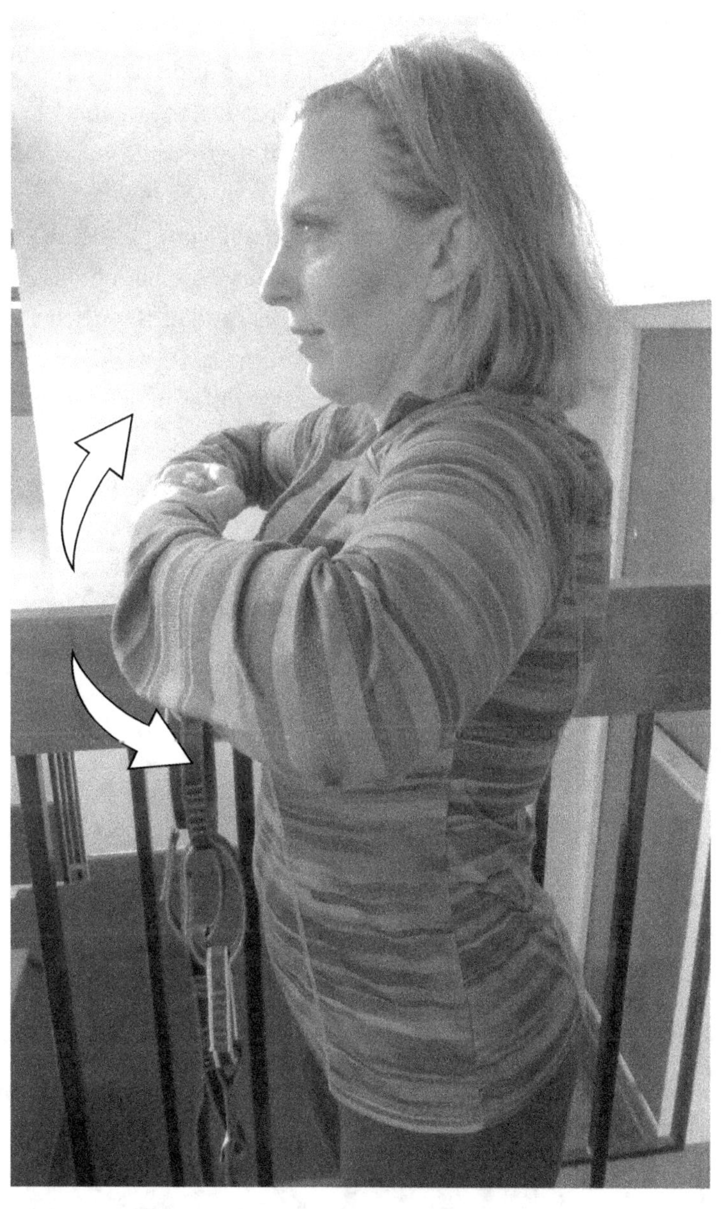

Section 4 Upper Back:

Overhead Upper-Back Pull-Apart

In either a seated or a standing position with your torso upright, raise your bent arms directly above your head. Your arms should be approximately vertical. Hold one loop of a daisy chain in both hands directly above your head. In this position, apply tension to pull your hands apart. Your grip on the loop prevents this from happening as you engage the upper back, shoulder, and neck muscles. An advanced user would also perform the same exercise with wider loops to exercise the back at different points on the ROM, or Range of Motion. When you perform an isometric exercise, never hold your breath. Always breathe deeply and naturally, which will be about 10 full breaths at a rate of about 1 second per breath. Perform each exercise for no less than 7 seconds and no longer than 10.

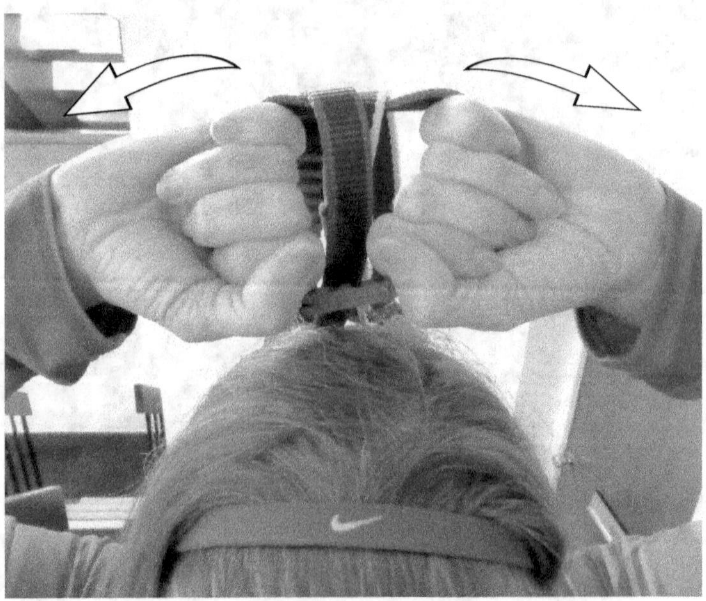

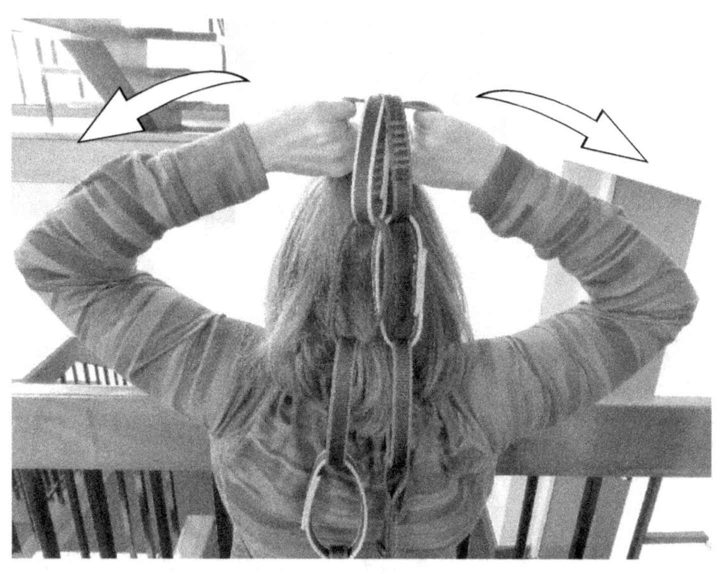

Below: Variation With Two Loops

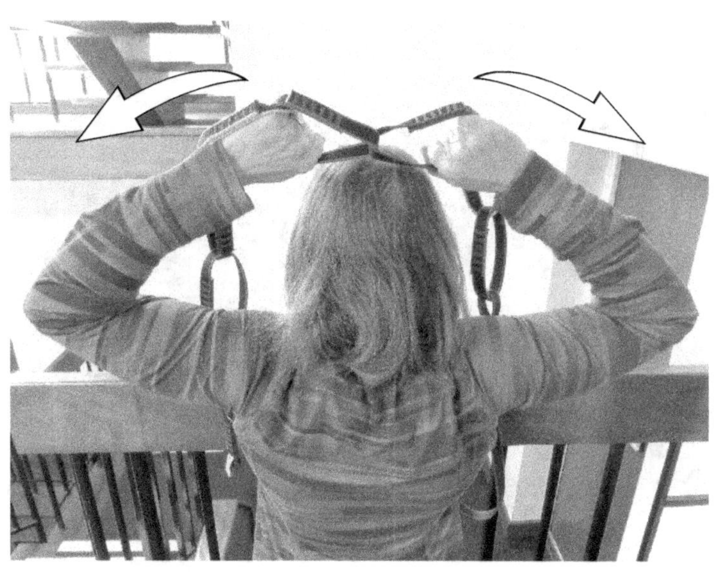

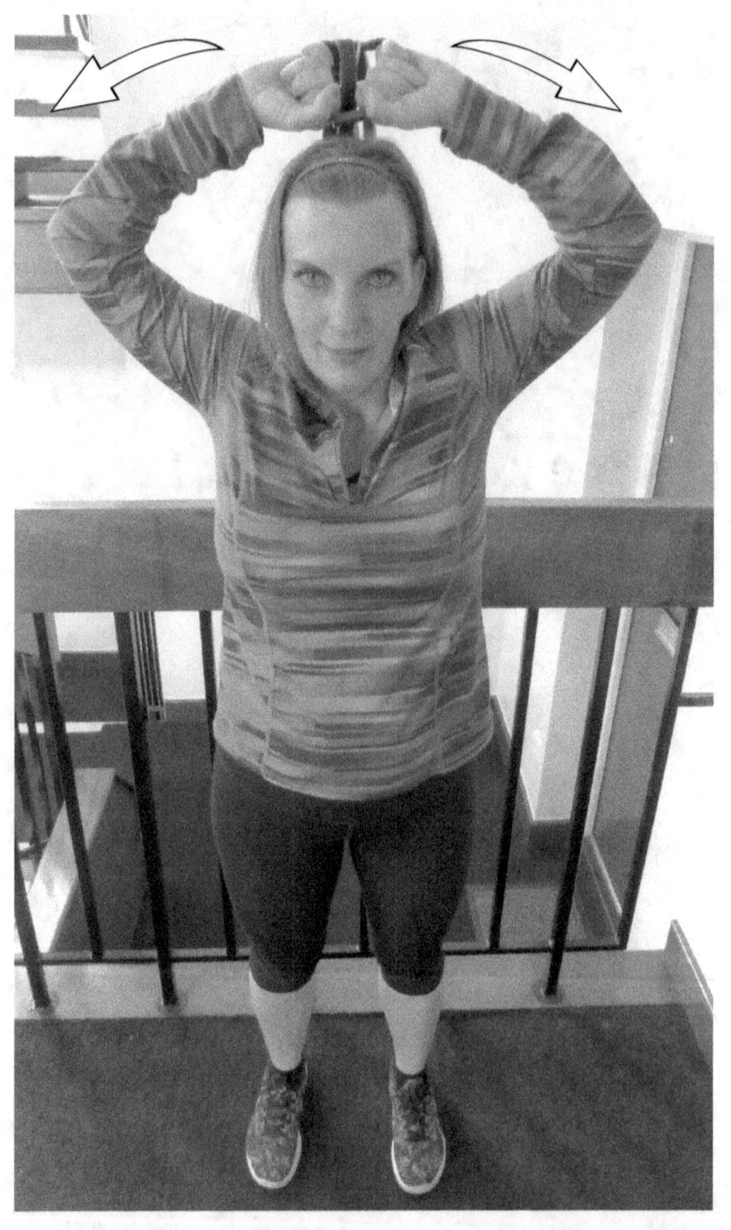

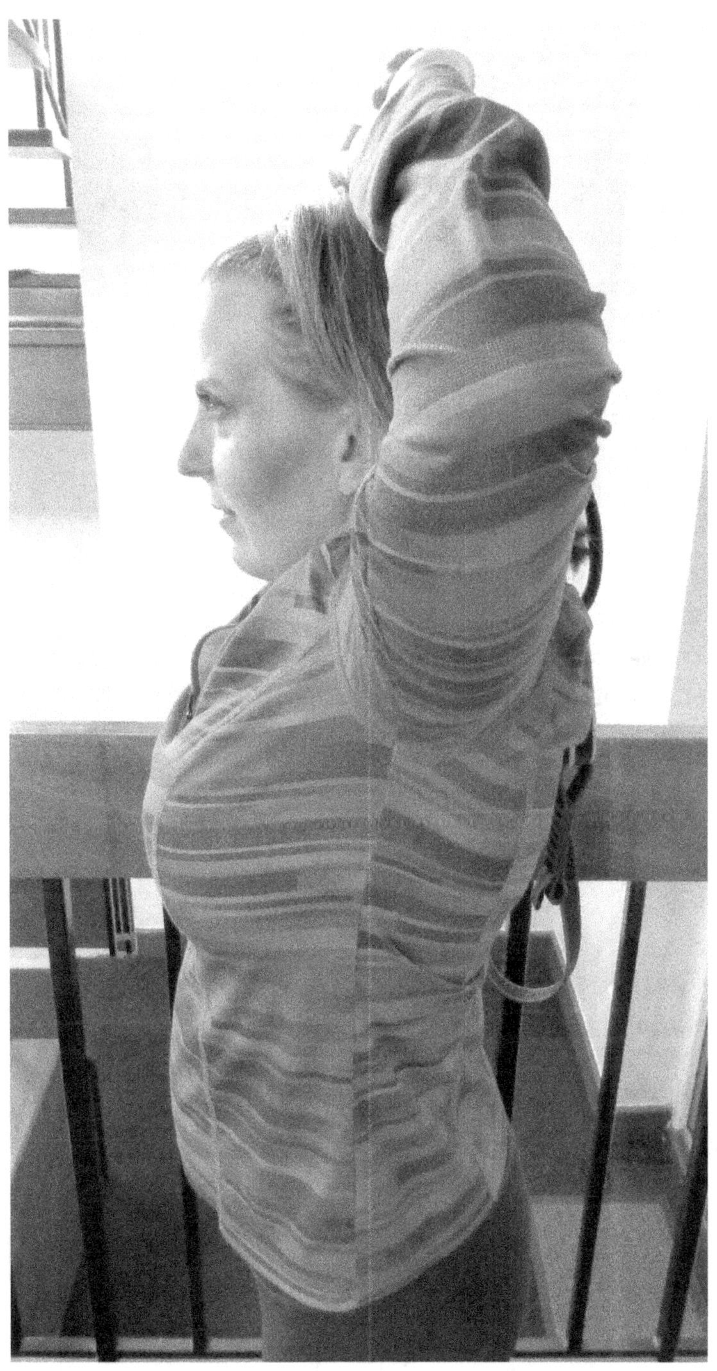

140

Section 4 Upper Back:

Seated Row

Either sit on the floor or a solid bench, then extend both legs forward. Secure the foot loop of each daisy chain around each foot. Bend your knees slightly and take hold of the same colour loop on each daisy chain, one in each hand. Keep your arms and elbows close to your body. In this position, apply tension to pull your hands backwards. Your grip on the loops prevents this from happening as you engage the upper back, shoulder, and neck muscles. Be sure to pull your arms backwards with your elbows leading the way to fully engage the upper back muscles and prevent the arm muscles from being the primary drivers. An advanced user would perform the same exercise with other loops as well. This will exercise the back at different points on the ROM, or Range of Motion. When you perform an isometric exercise, never hold your breath. Always breathe deeply and naturally, which will be about 10 full breaths at a rate of about 1 second per breath. Perform each exercise for no less than 7 seconds and no longer than 10.

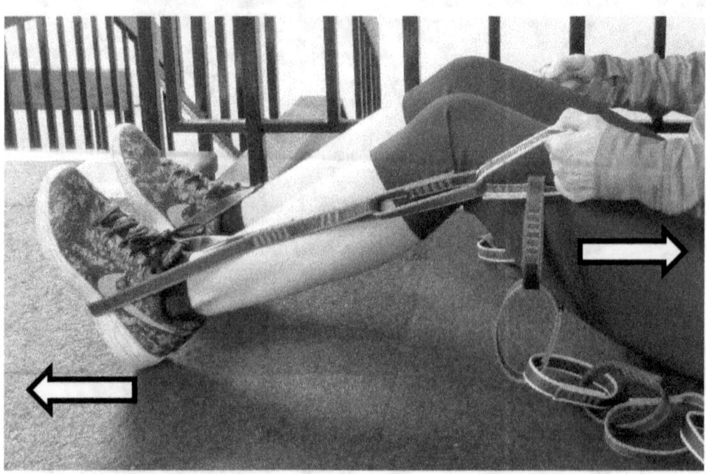

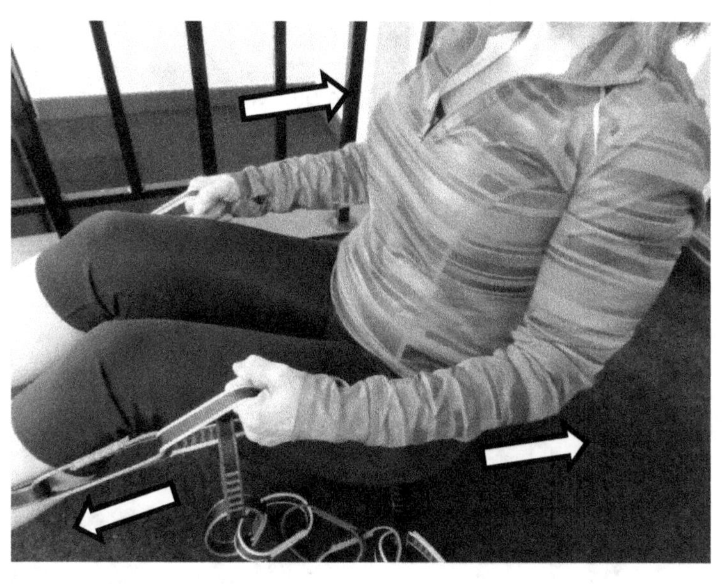

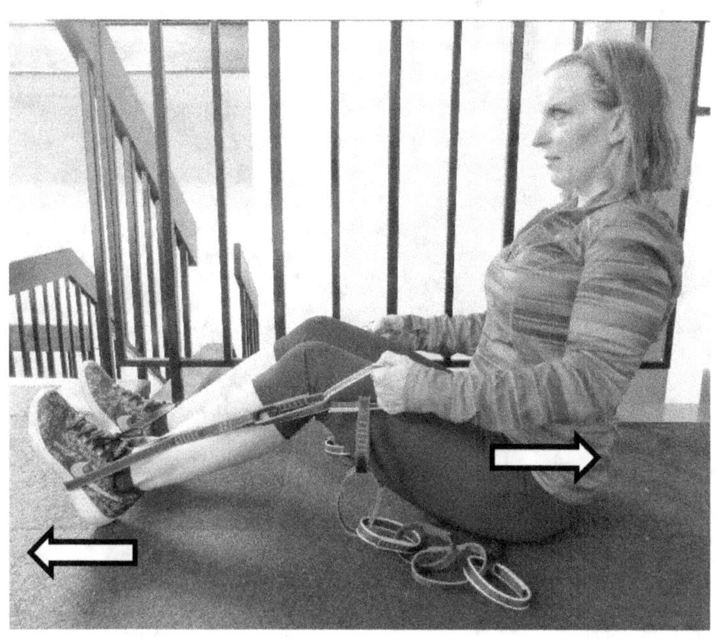

Below: Variation With Bench

The seated row variation below, using a bench, will shift the focus of the exercise to a slightly higher part of the upper back, depending upon how high the seated position is. The lower the feet, the higher the focus, and vice versa.

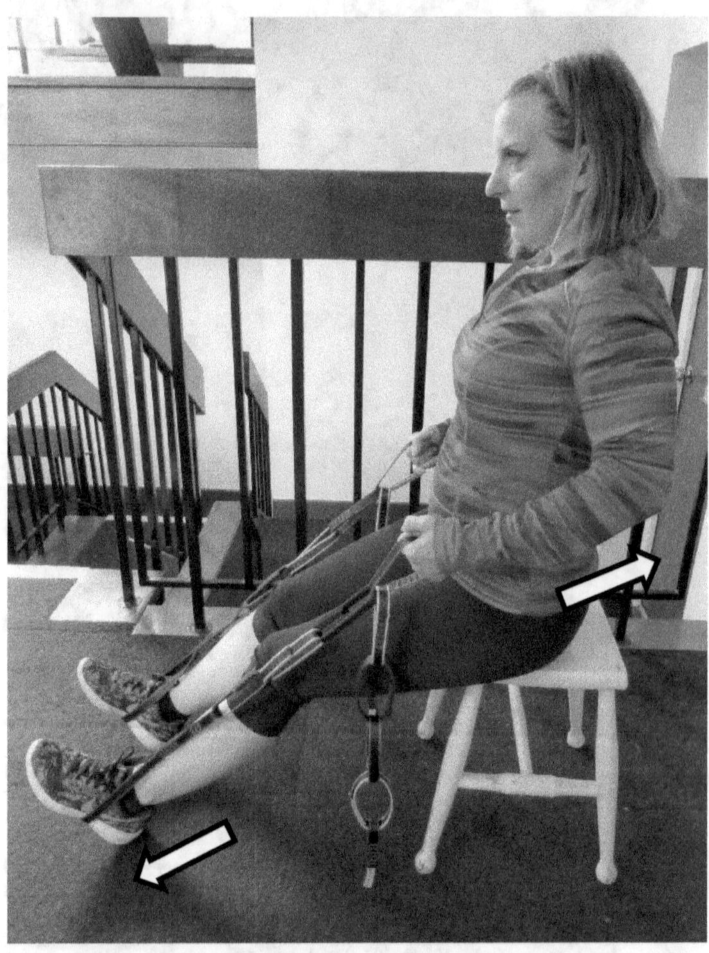

Section 4 Upper Back:

Standing Single Arm Row

Stand with one foot forward in a high semi-lunge position and place the foot loop of a daisy chain around the leading foot. Bend forward slightly, only from the hips and keep your back straight. Take hold of a daisy chain loop that allows you to perform a general exercise with the arm bent at approximately 90 degrees. Pull your arms backwards with your elbows leading the way to fully engage the upper back muscles and prevent the arm muscles from being the primary drivers. An advanced user would also perform the same exercise with other loops to exercise the back at different points on the ROM, or Range of Motion. It is OK to hold onto a bench or any other solid object with the other hand to aid your stability. When you perform an isometric exercise, never hold your breath. Always breathe deeply and naturally, which will be about 10 full breaths at a rate of about 1 second per breath. Perform each exercise for no less than 7 seconds and no longer than 10.

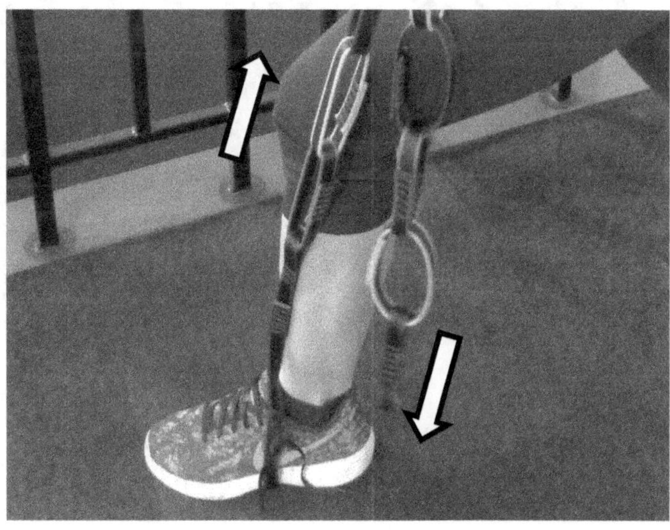

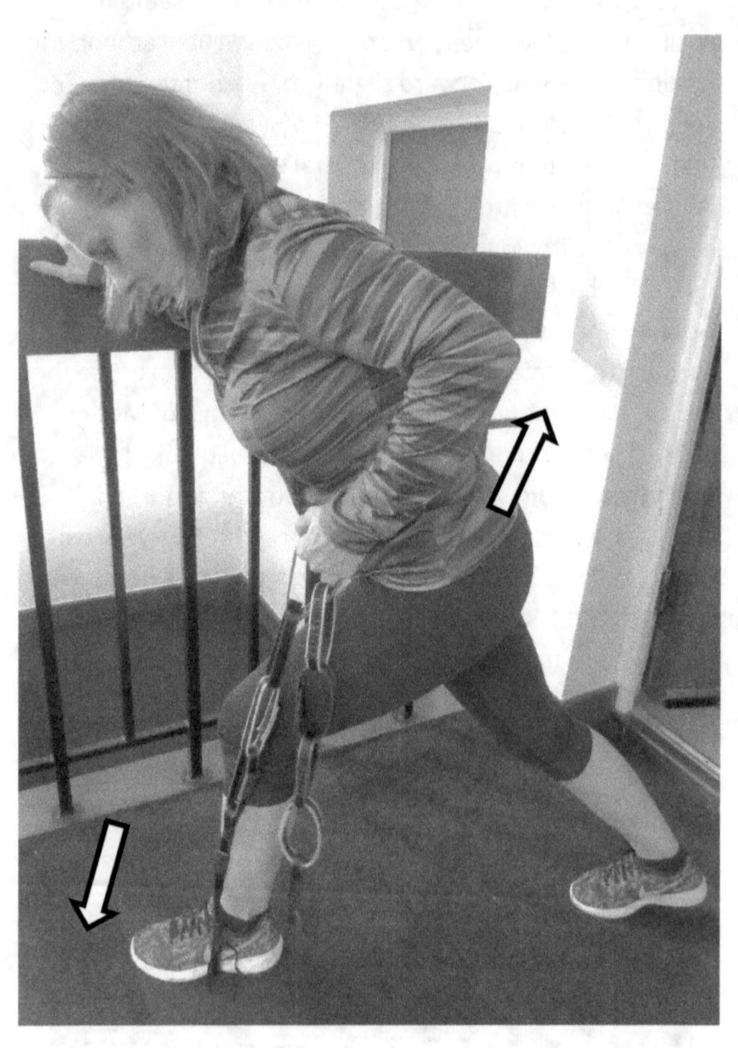

Section 5 Lower Back:

Good Morning Overhead Pull-Apart

Stand upright with your feet approximately shoulder-width apart. Bend forward from the hips, keeping your back straight, until your torso is approximately horizontal to the floor. Extend both arms shoulder-width apart straight above your head while holding a daisy chain in both hands. Pull the daisy chain apart and, at the same time, engage the lower and mid-back muscles to support you during the exercise. When you perform an isometric exercise, never hold your breath. Always breathe deeply and naturally, which will be about 10 full breaths at a rate of about 1 second per breath. Perform each exercise for no less than 7 seconds and no longer than 10.

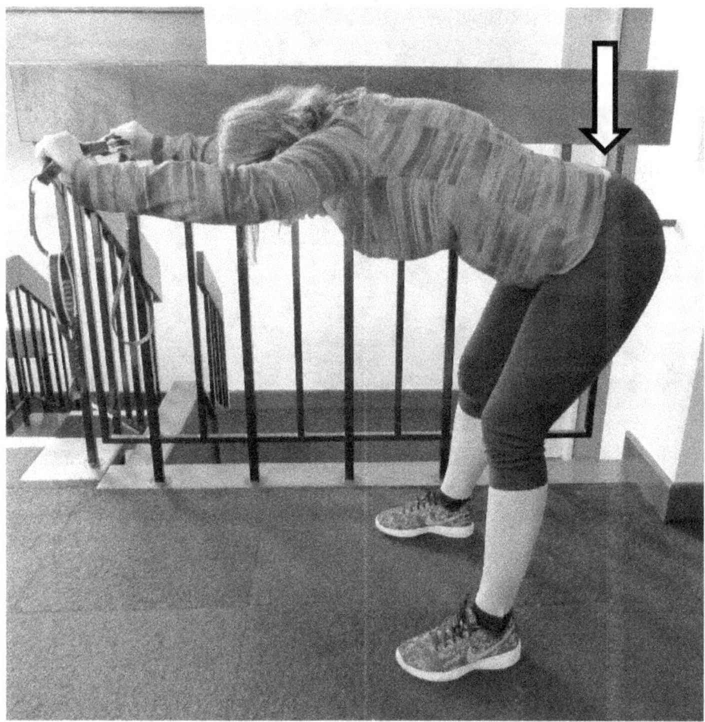

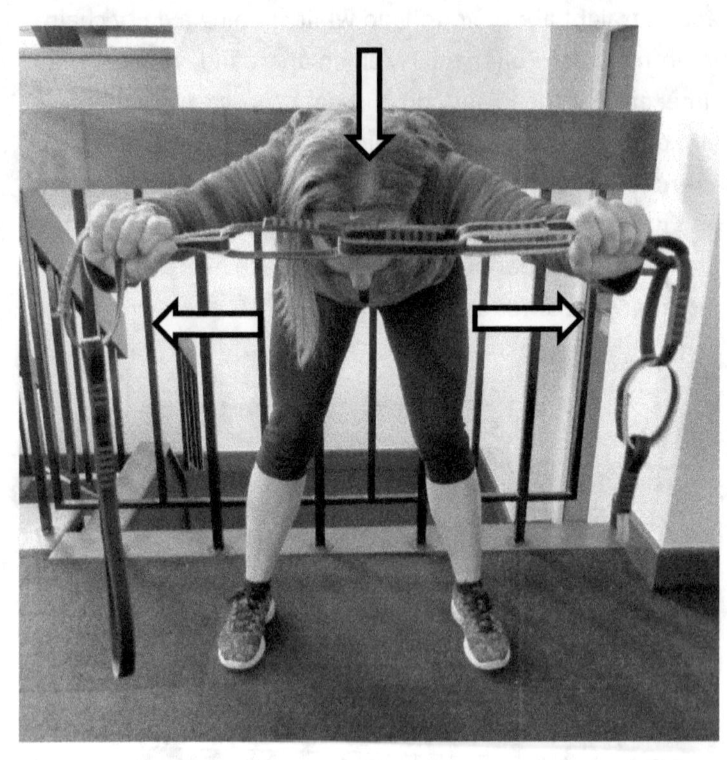

Section 5 Lower Back:

The Deadlift

Stand with your feet roughly shoulder-width apart, with one foot in each of the foot loops of a pair of daisy chains. Select a hand loop of the same colour on each side that will allow you to perform the deadlift at your angle of choice for a general lower back exercise. As you squat slightly, bend forward from the hips and keep your back straight. Grip the loop, and, using your lower back muscles and glutes as the primary drivers, lift into a deadlift position to perform the exercise. Advanced users may wish to use several different loop positions to perform the deadlift exercise at different points on the ROM – Range of Motion of the exercise. When you perform an isometric exercise, never hold your breath. Always breathe deeply and naturally, which will be about 10 full breaths at a rate of about 1 second per breath. Perform each exercise for no less than 7 seconds and no longer than 10 seconds.

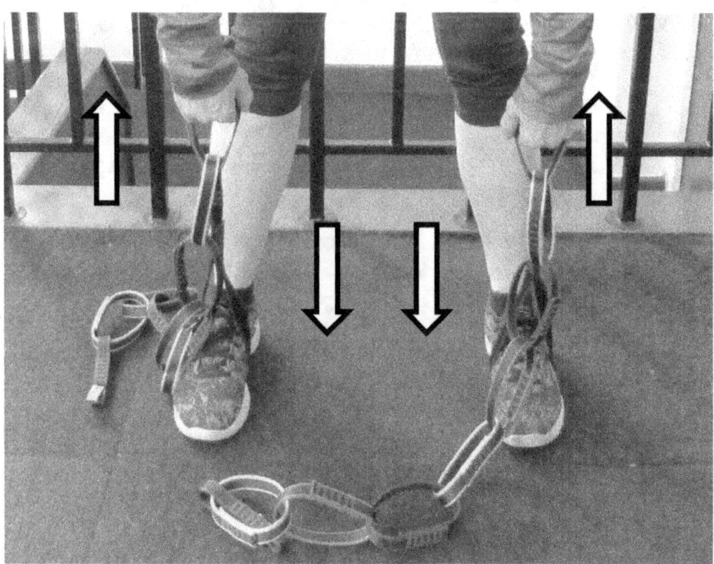

148

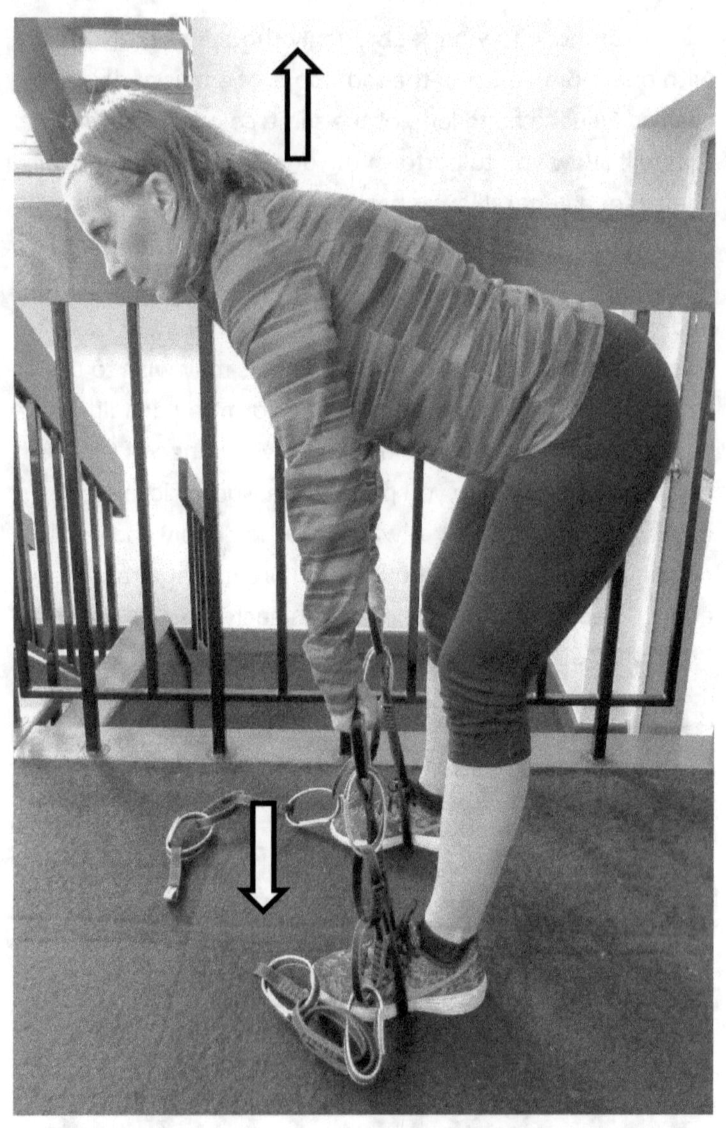

149

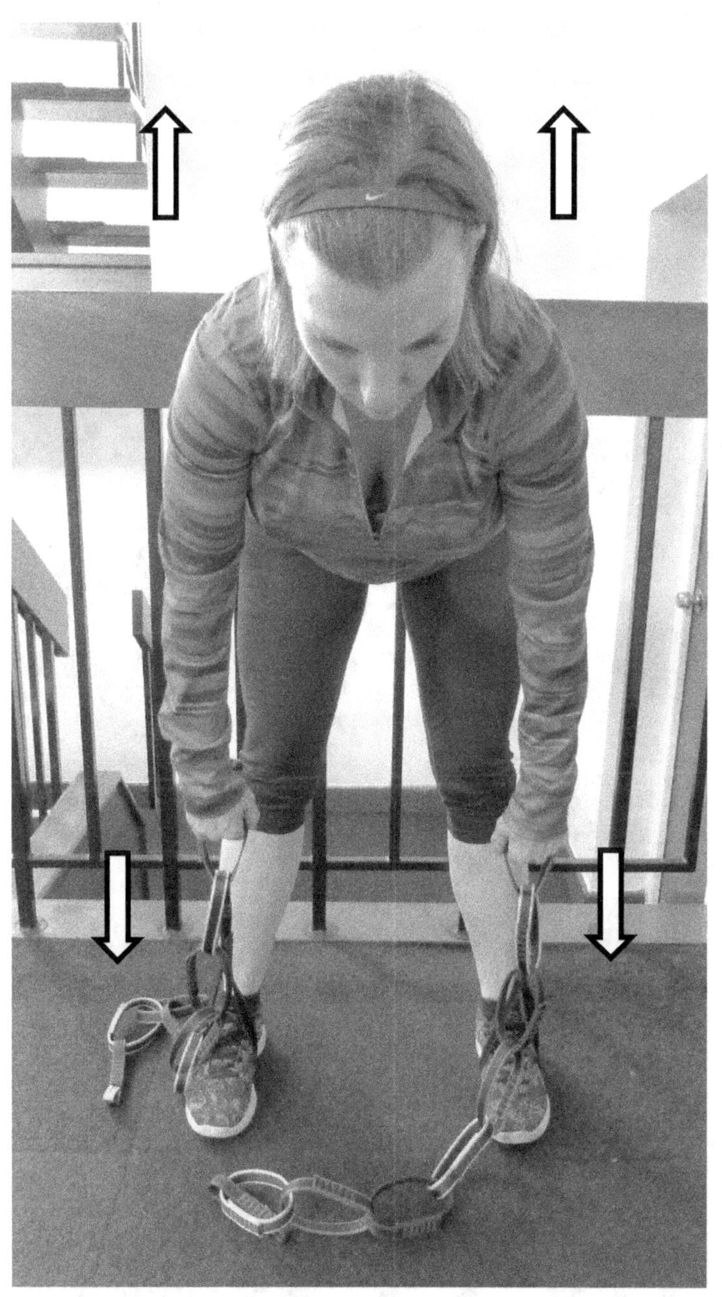

150

Variation in a Higher Deadlift Position

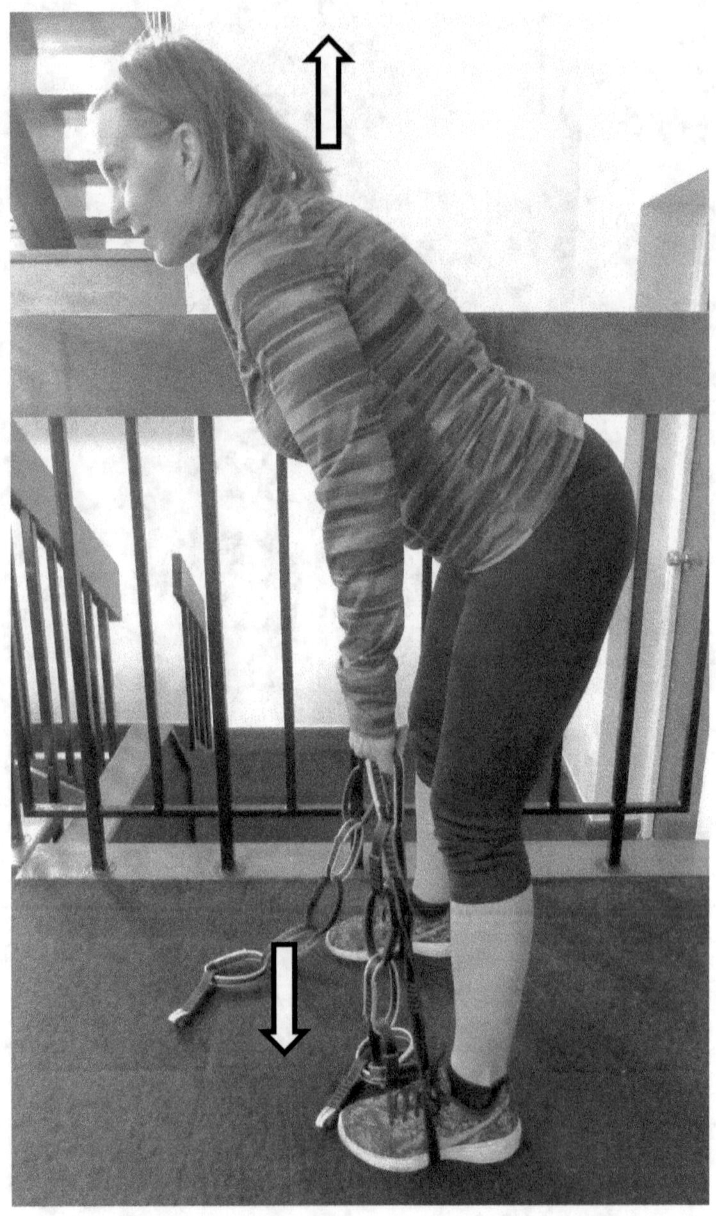

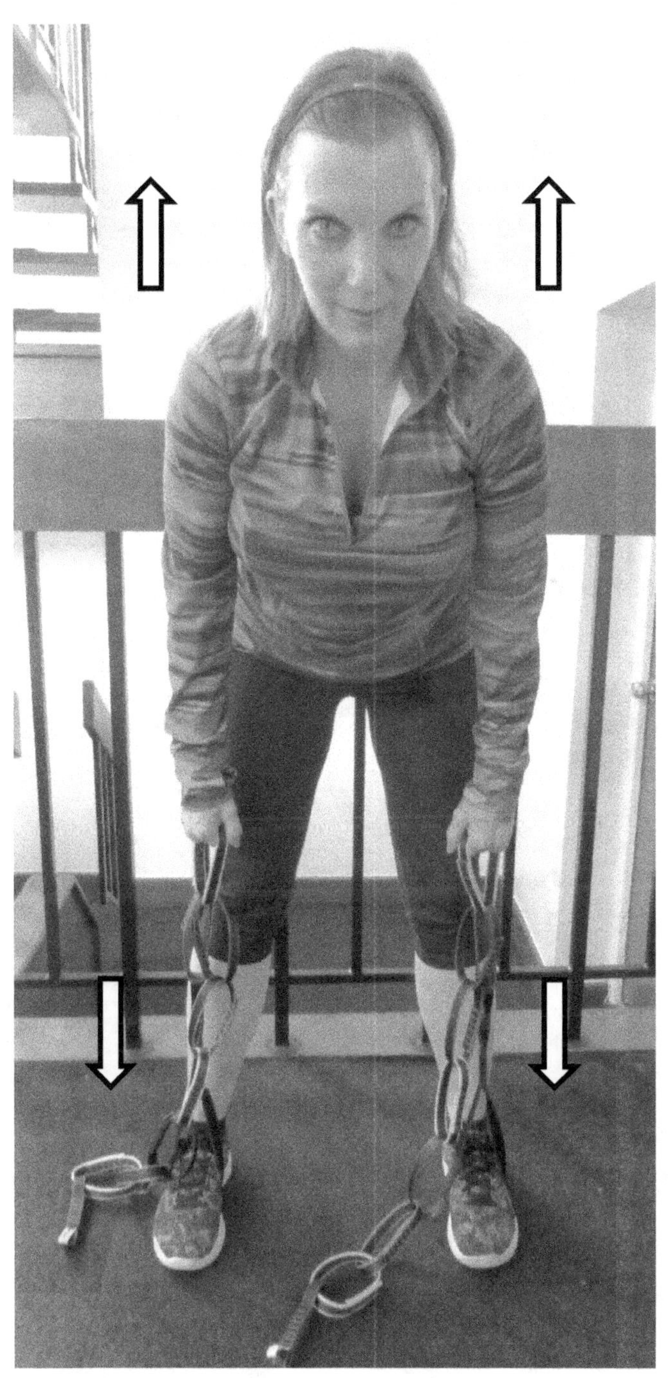

Section 6 Chest:

Chest Cross-Press

In either a seated or standing position, firmly grip one approximately central loop of a single daisy chain. Allow your hands to slightly cross past each other as you press across your chest.

Ensure that your elbows and arms are out and to the side so your upper arms are approximately parallel to the floor. In this position, using the chest muscles as the primary drivers, increase the force as you press your hands across your chest with the loop resisting you to perform the exercise.

When you perform an isometric exercise, never hold your breath. Always breathe deeply and naturally, which will be about 10 full breaths at a rate of about 1 second per breath.   Perform each exercise for no less than 7 seconds and no longer than 10.

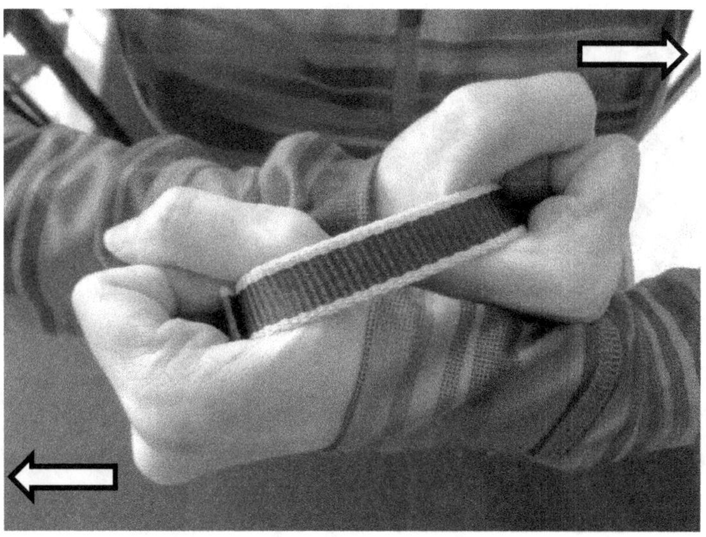

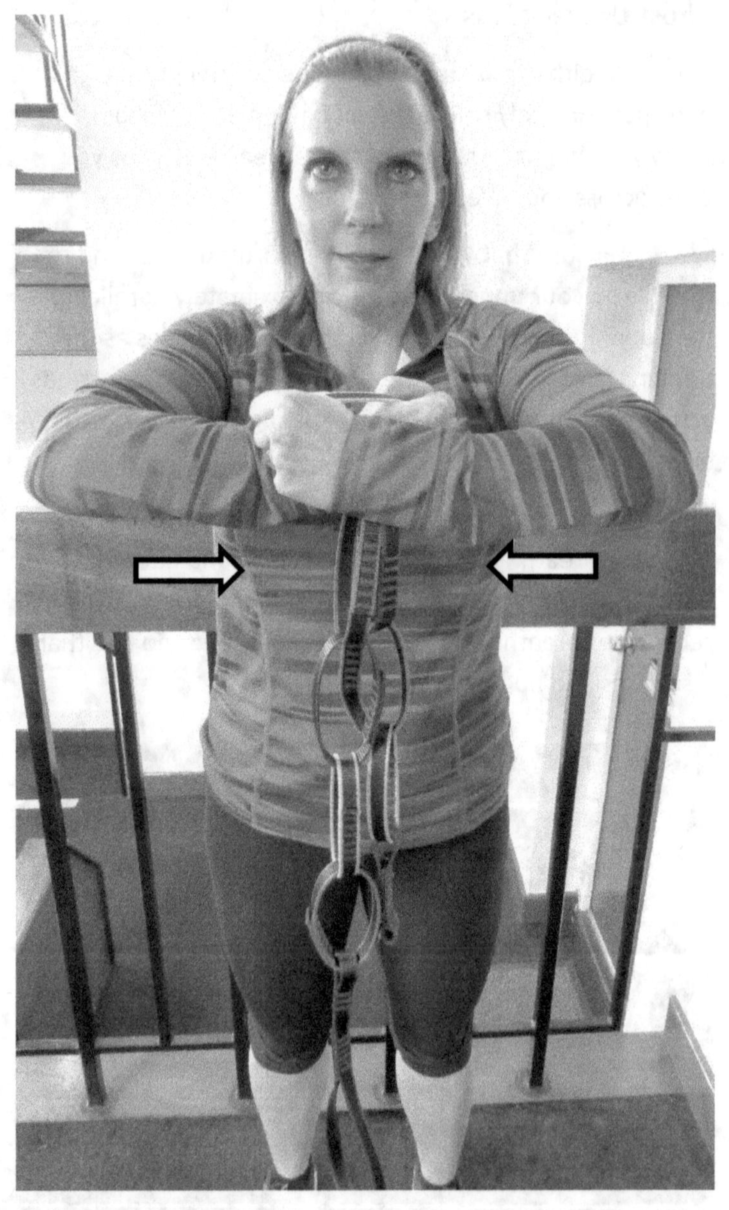

155

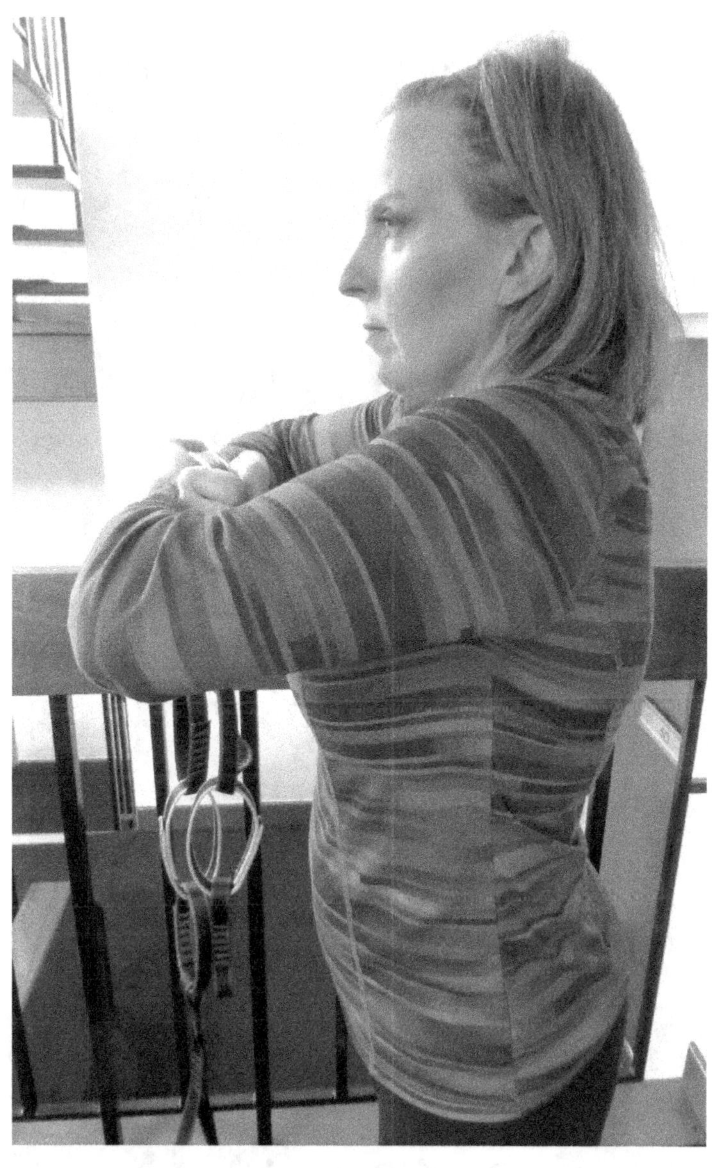

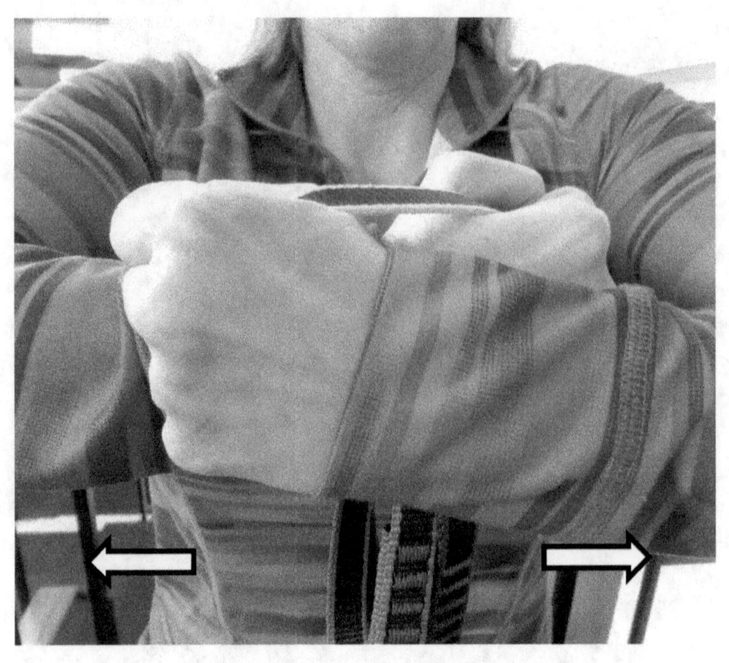

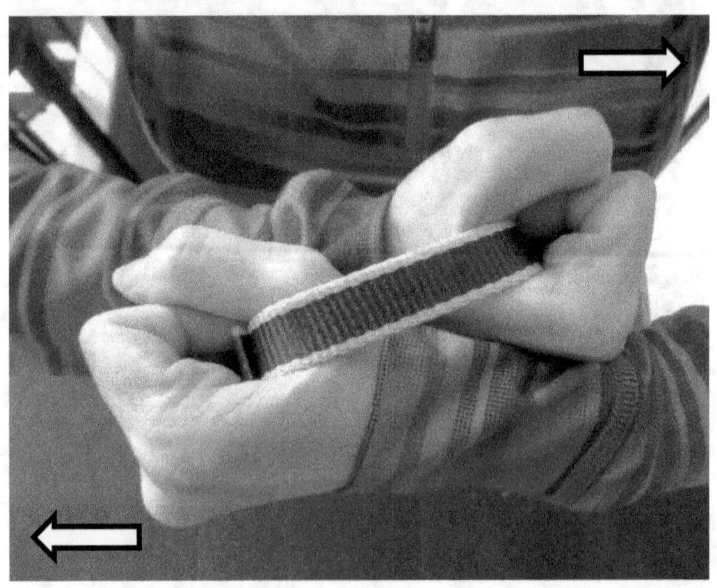

Section 6 Chest:

Across Back Flye

Place a daisy chain evenly across your back so that
the ends fall across your shoulders. Grip an appropriately
positioned loop at each end. Ensure that your elbows and
arms are out and to the side so your upper arms are
approximately parallel to the floor. Using the chest muscles
as the primary drivers, increase the force as you press your
hands inwards and slightly forward across your chest. The
loops will then prevent you from performing the chest flye
exercise. When you perform an isometric exercise, never
hold your breath. Always breathe deeply and naturally,
which will be about 10 full breaths at a rate of about 1
second per breath.   Perform each exercise for no less than
7 seconds and no longer than 10.

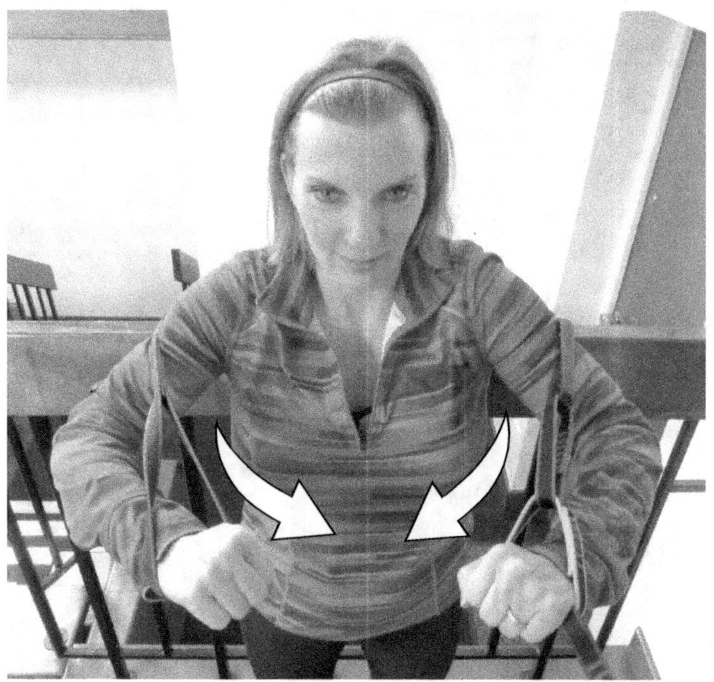

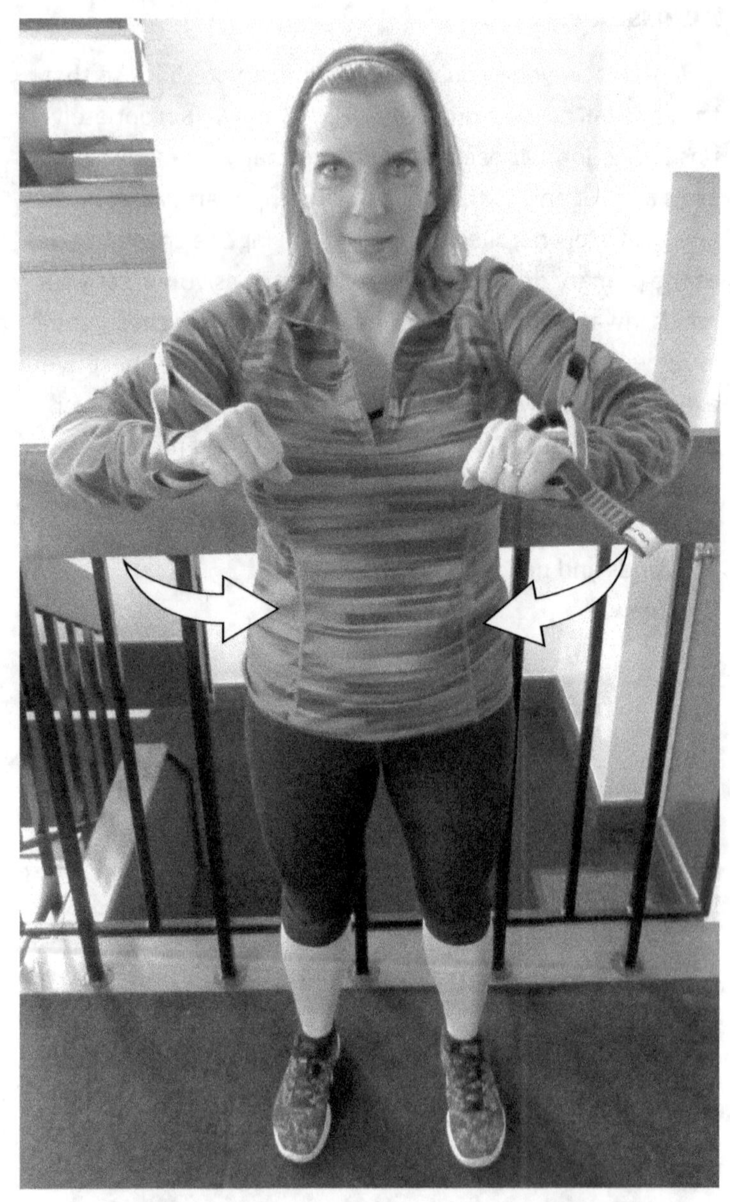

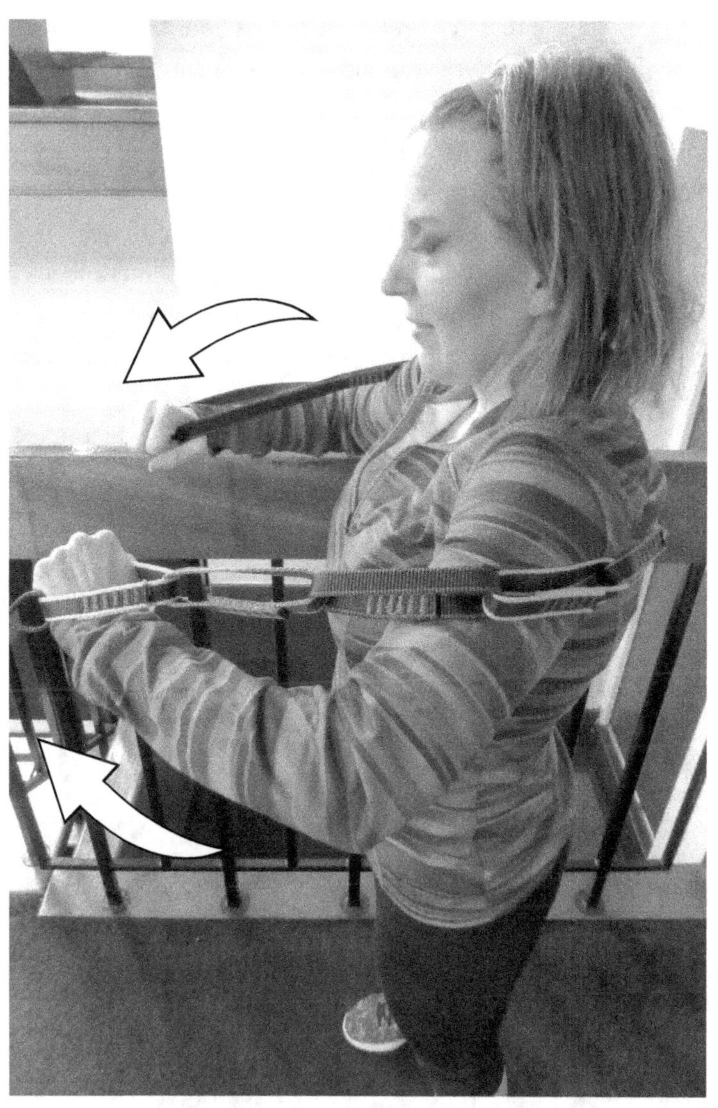

Section 6 Chest:

Standing Chest Press

Place a daisy chain evenly across your back so that the ends fall across your shoulders. Grip an appropriately positioned loop at each end. Ensure that your upper arms are out and to the side and approximately parallel to the floor with your elbows bent at an approximate angle of 90 degrees. Using the chest muscles as the primary drivers, increase the force as you press your hands forward and very slightly inward, with the loops resisting you from performing the standing chest press exercise.

When you perform an isometric exercise, never hold your breath. Always breathe deeply and naturally, which will be about 10 full breaths at a rate of about 1 second per breath. Perform each exercise for no less than 7 seconds and no longer than 10.

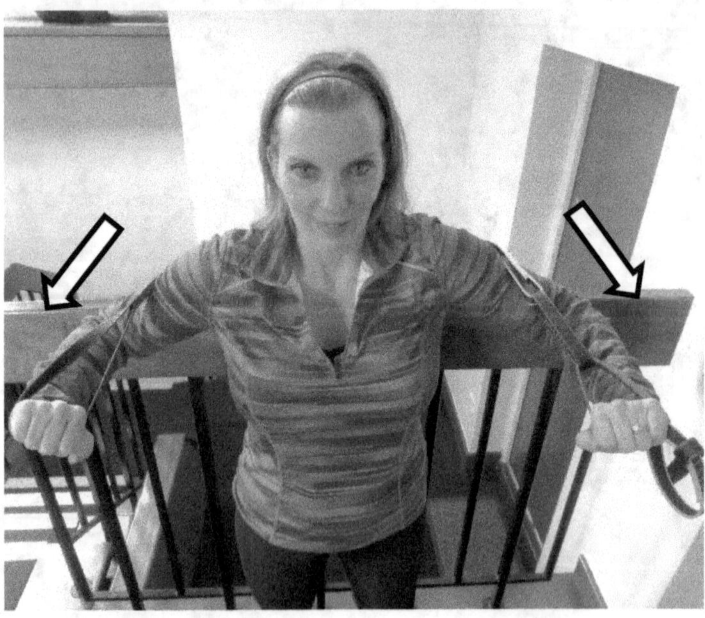

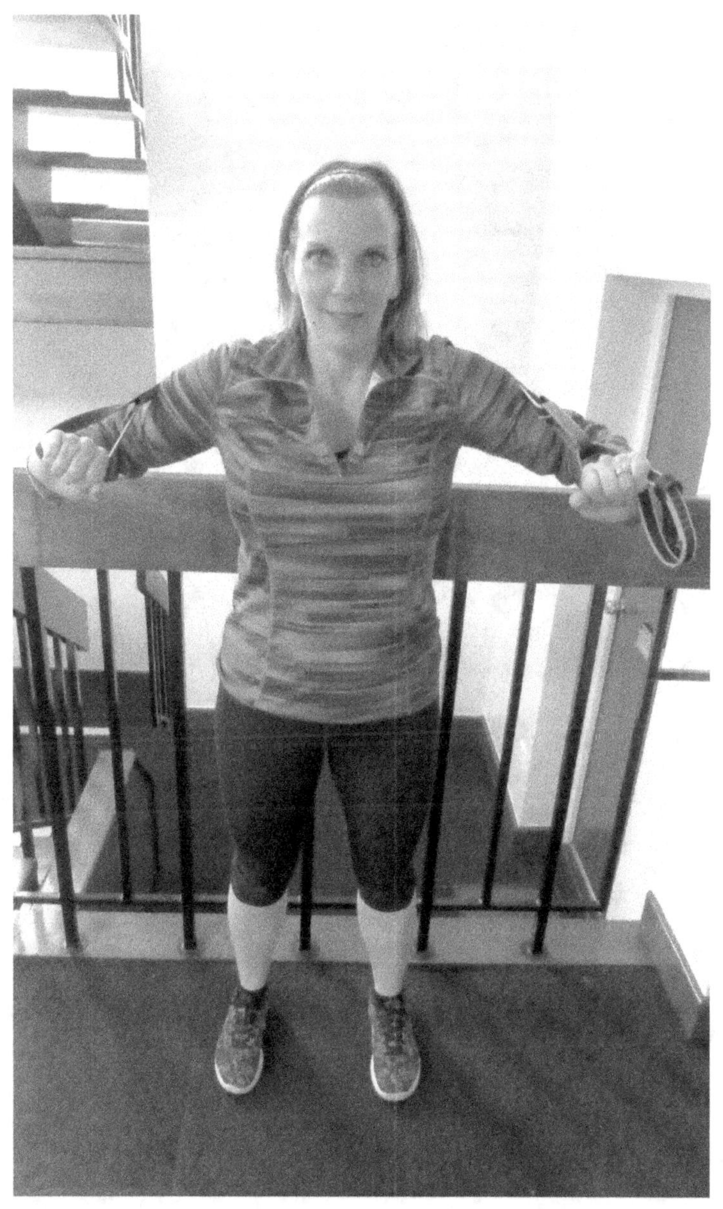

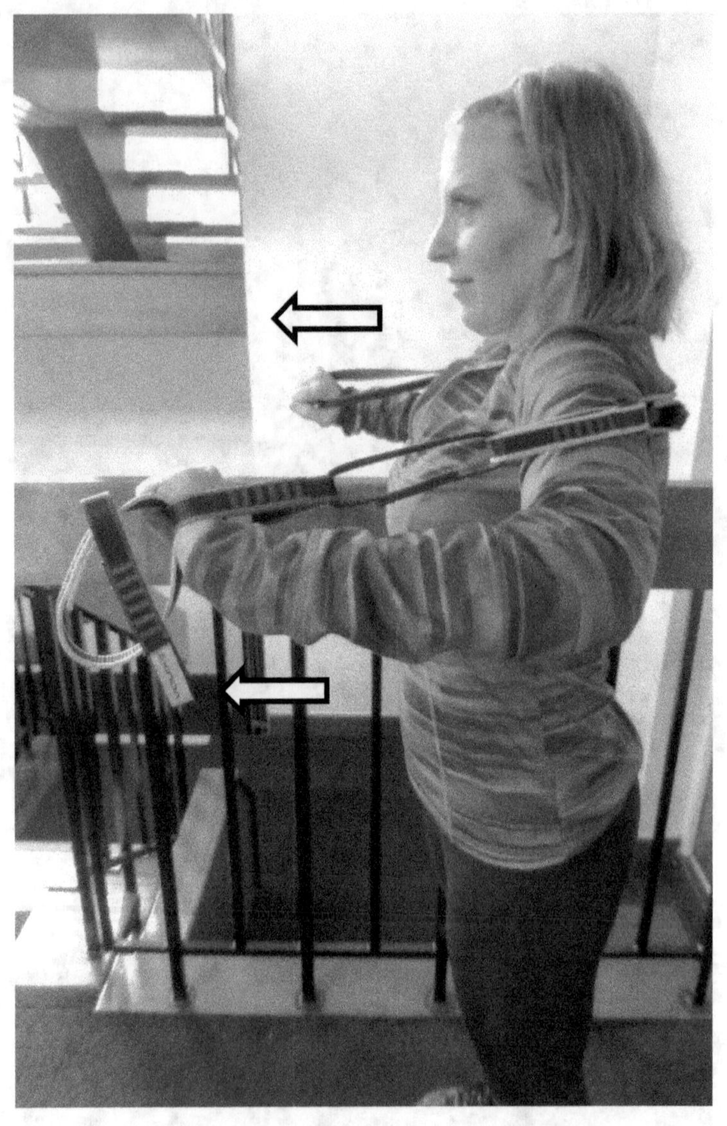

Section 6 Chest:

Resisted Push-up

Lying face-down in the push-up position on the floor, place a daisy chain evenly across your upper back so that the ends fall on each side. Grip an appropriately positioned loop at each end. Ensure that your upper arms are out and to the side with your elbows bent at an approximate angle of 90 degrees. Using the chest muscles as the primary drivers, increase the force as you press your hands down and very slightly inwards with the loops resisting you to perform the resisted push-up exercise. When you perform an isometric exercise, never hold your breath. Always breathe deeply and naturally, which will be about 10 full breaths at a rate of about 1 second per breath. Perform each exercise for no less than 7 seconds and no longer than 10.

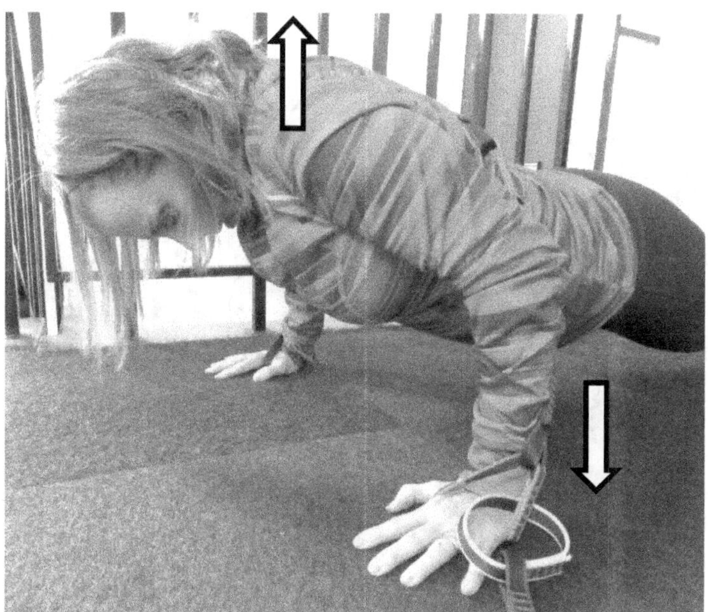

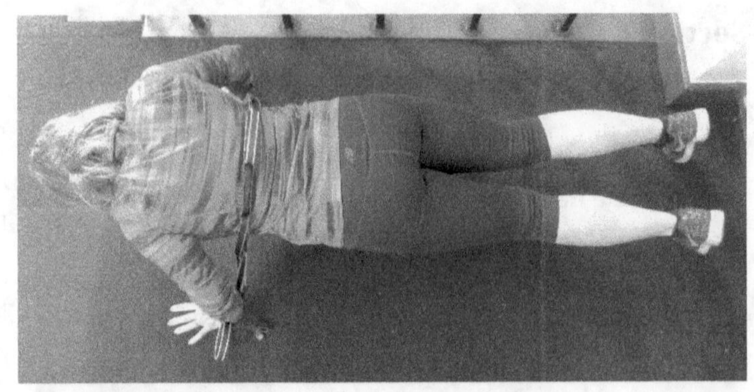

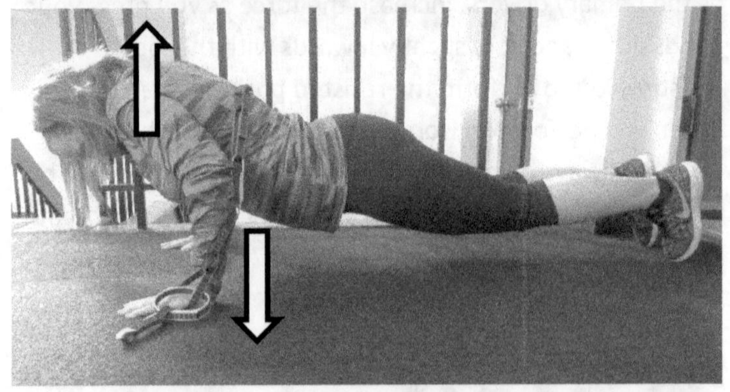

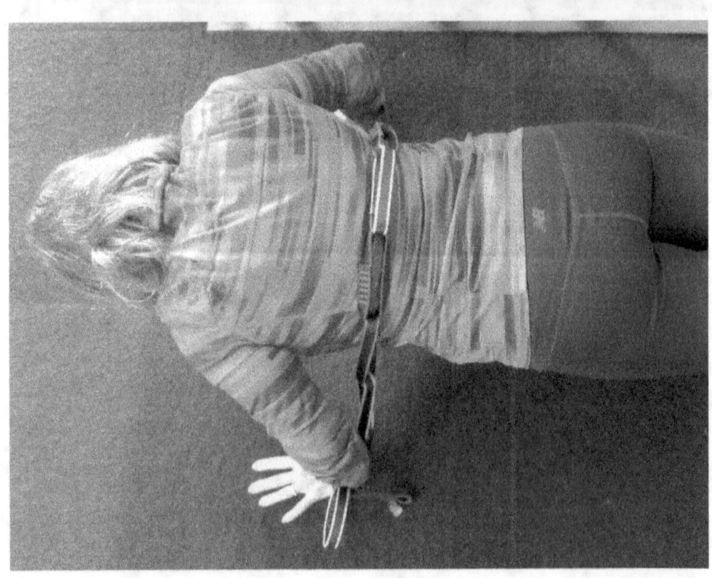

Section 7 Shoulders:

Side Lateral Raise

Stand upright and grip a single central loop of a daisy chain in front of you at arm's length. Bend both arms slightly at the elbow. Keep your arms and elbows locked in this position, and attempt to raise the arms sideways in an arcing move. Use your shoulder muscles as the driving force to perform the exercise. Advanced users may wish to use increasingly wider daisy chain loops to exercise the shoulders at different points on the ROM (Range of Motion) of the arms and shoulders.

When you perform an isometric exercise, never hold your breath. Always breathe deeply and naturally, which will be about 10 full breaths at a rate of about 1 second per breath.   Perform each exercise for no less than 7 seconds and no longer than 10.

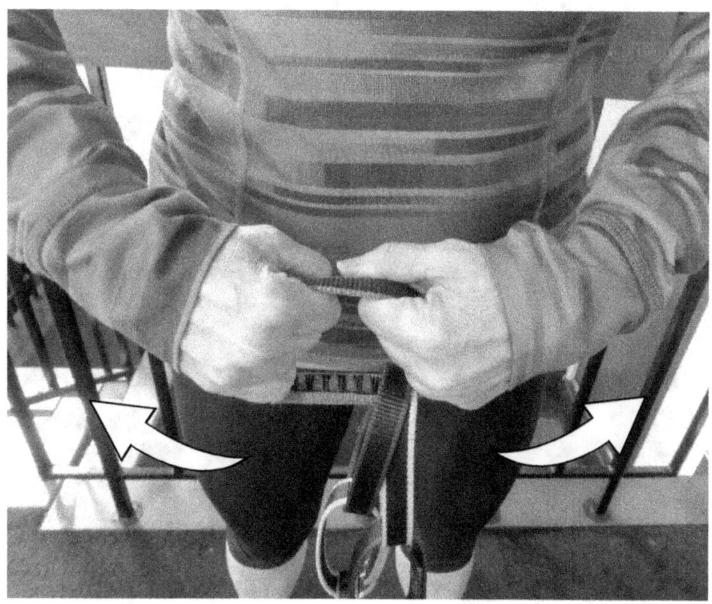

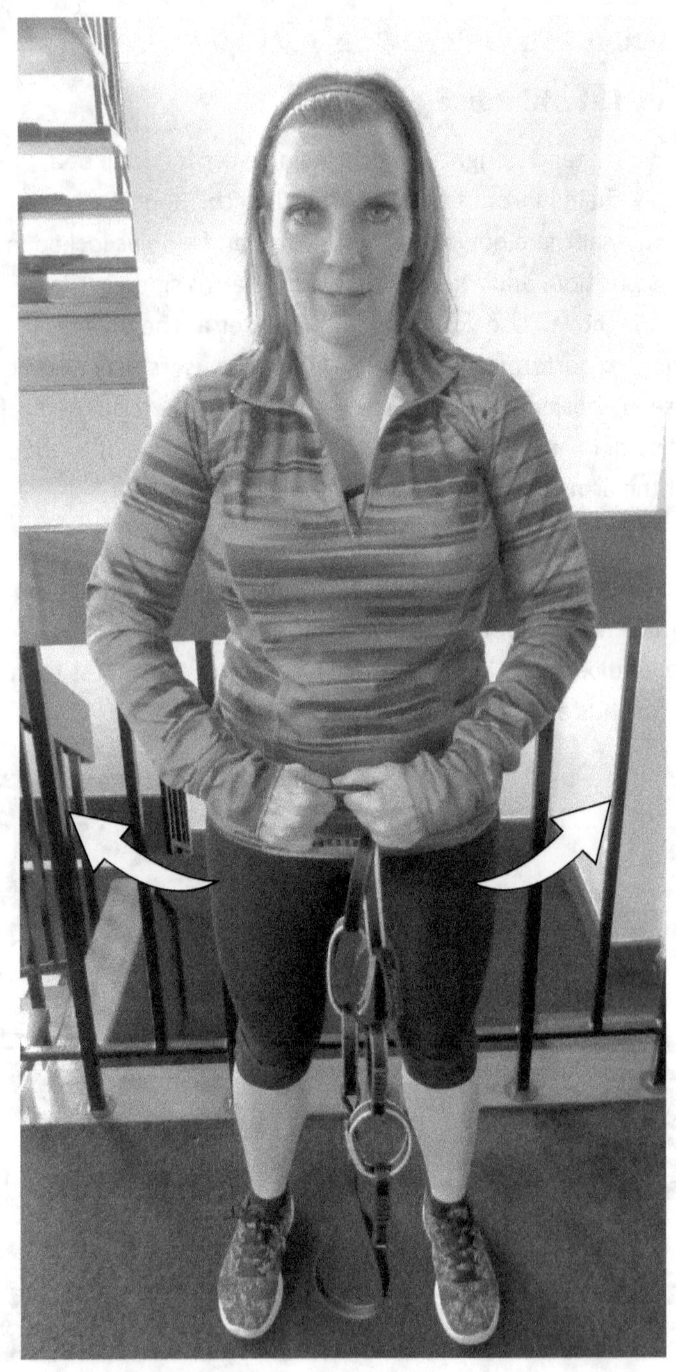

167

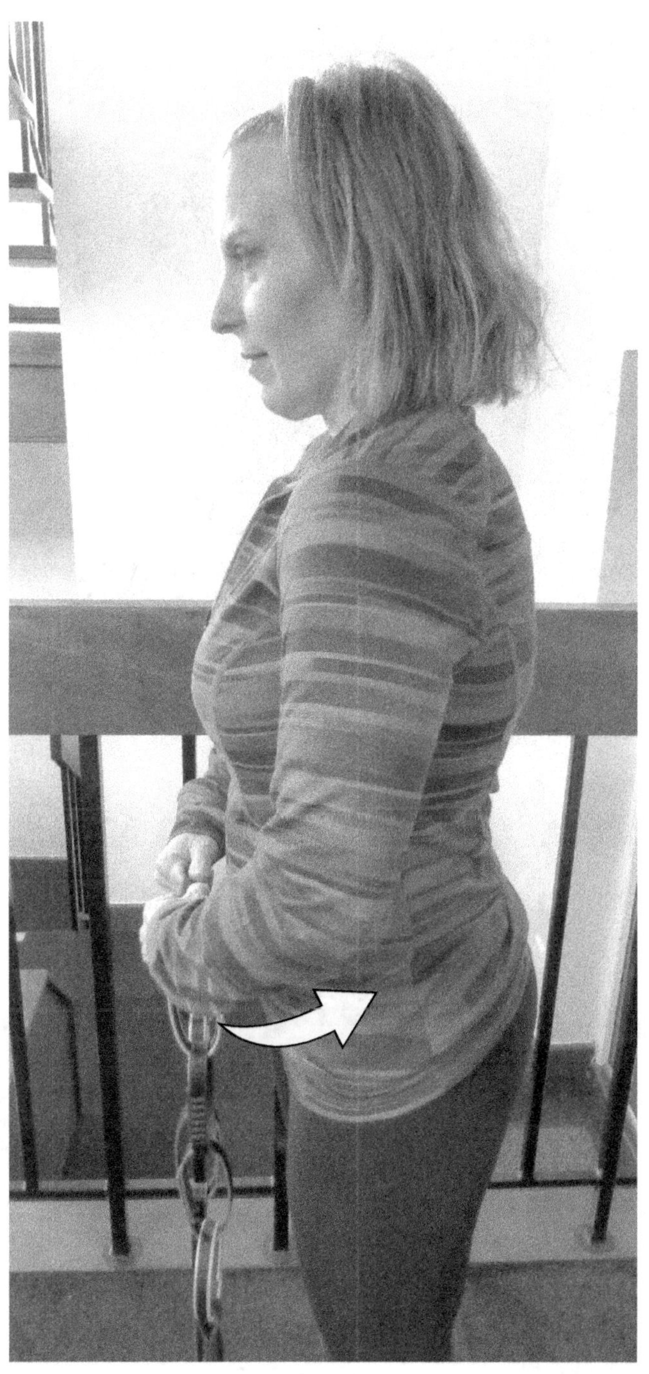

Section 7 Shoulders Variations:

Side Lateral Raise – Wider Loops

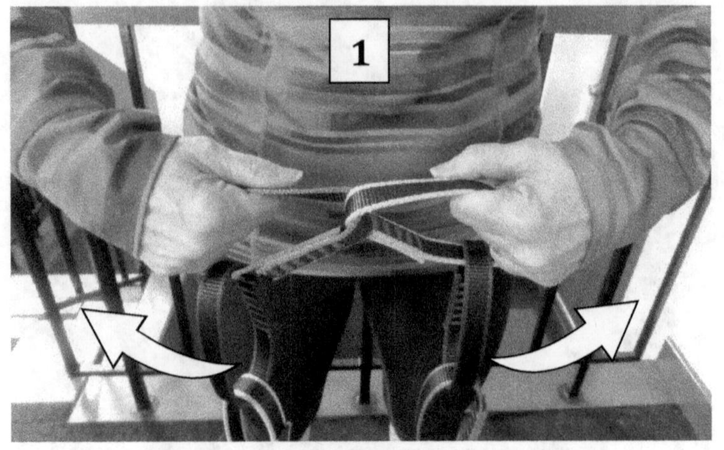

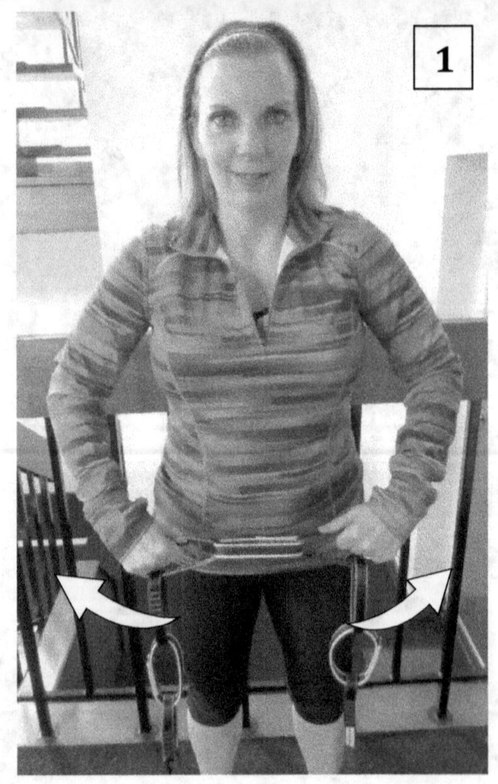

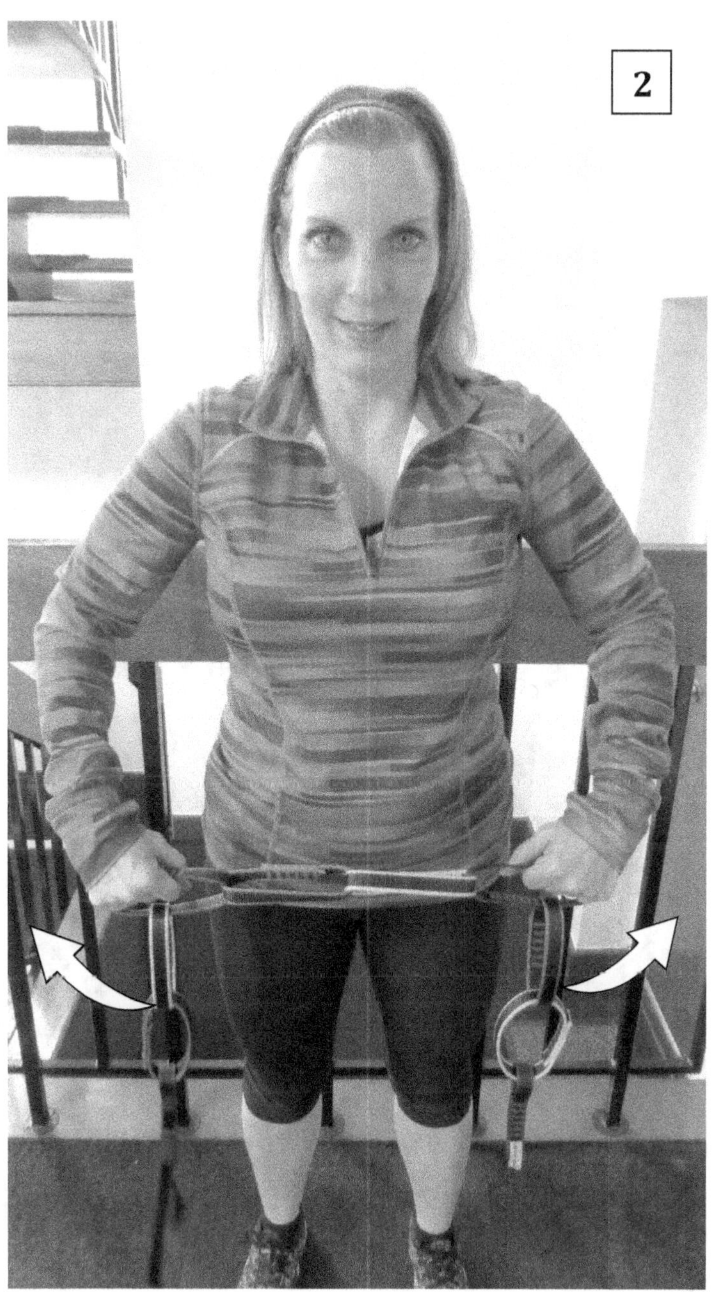

2

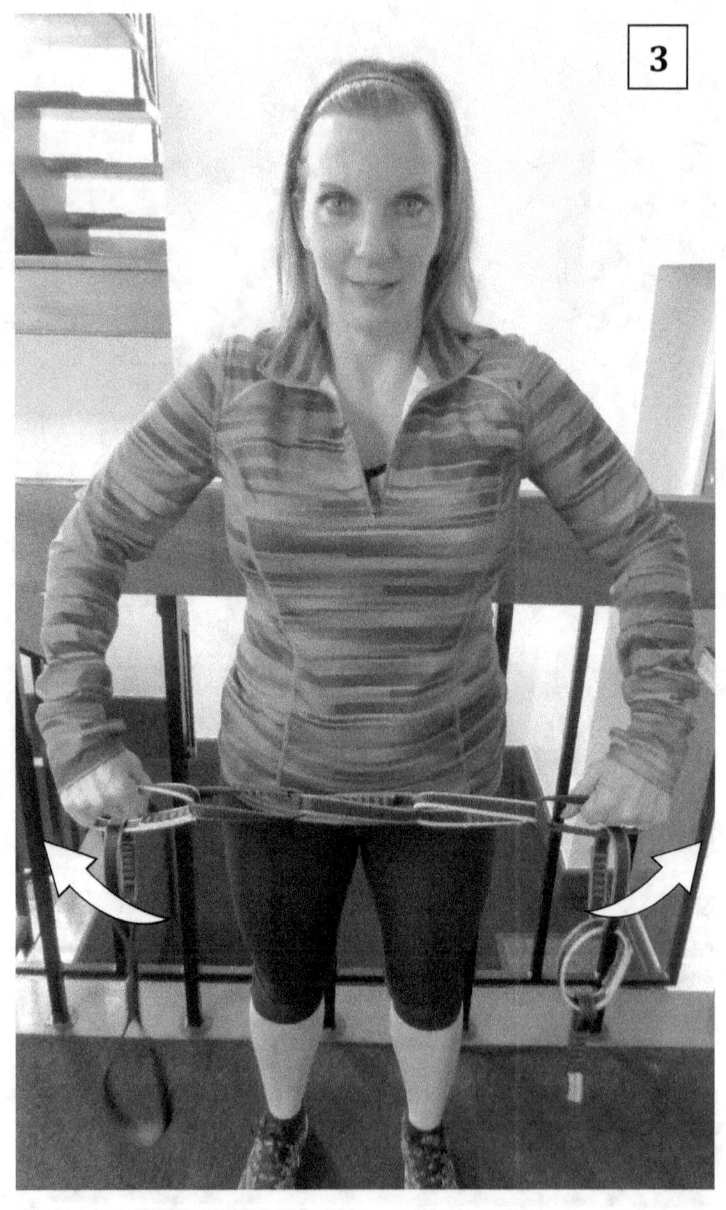

3

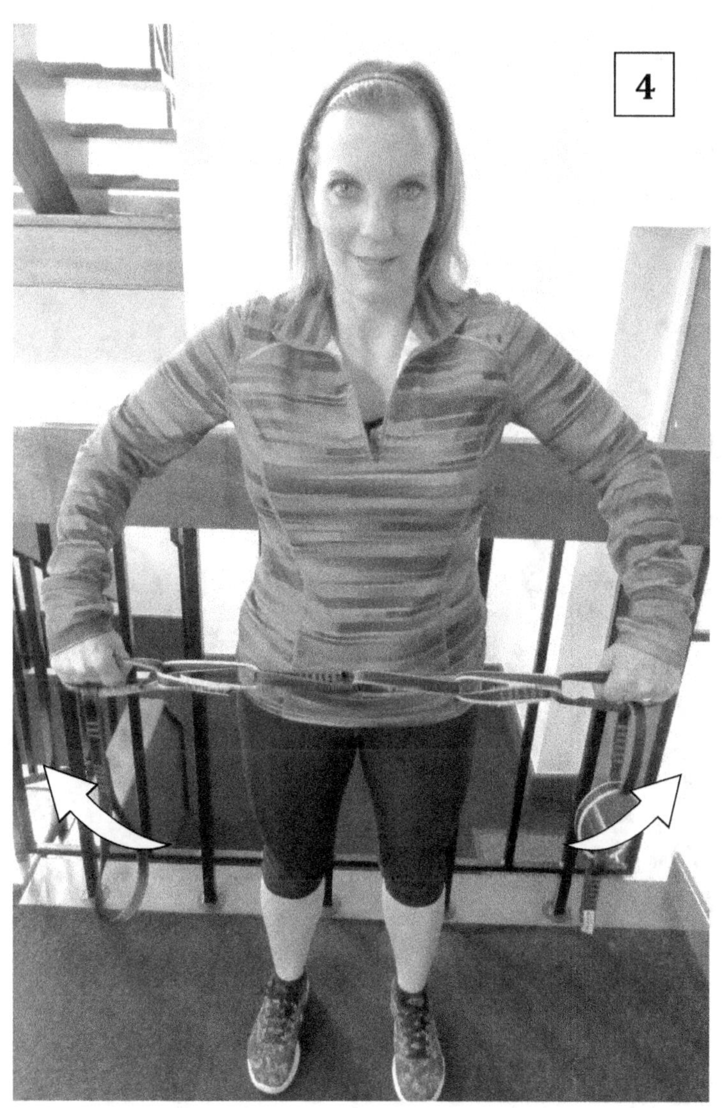

4

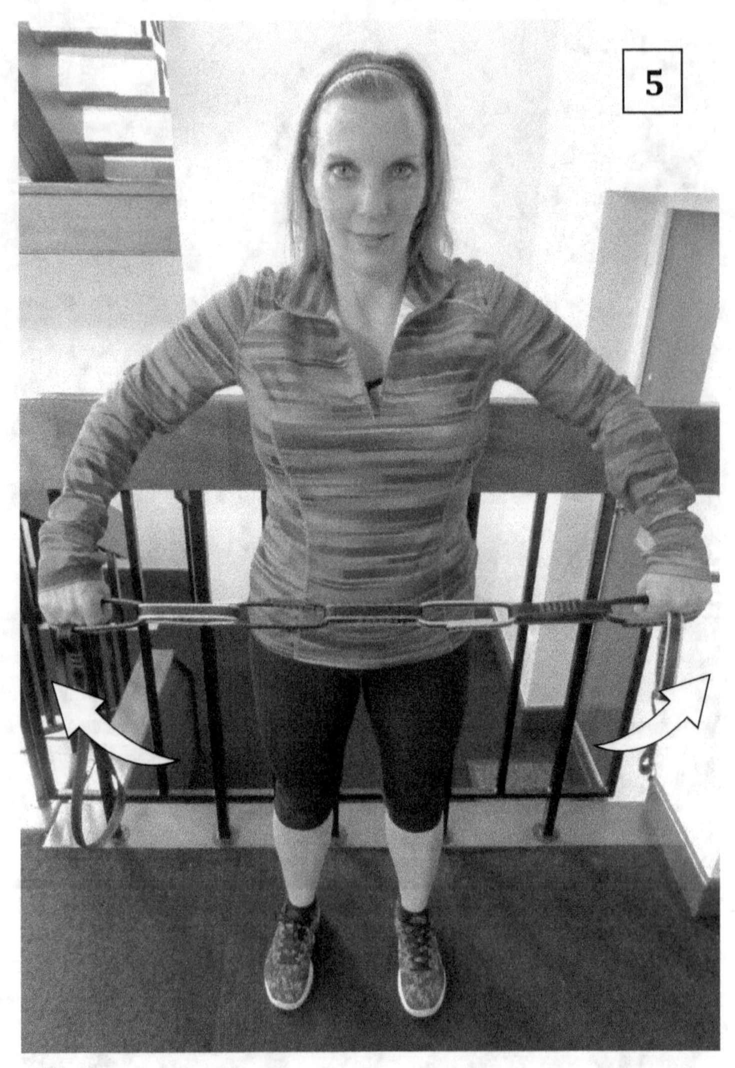

5

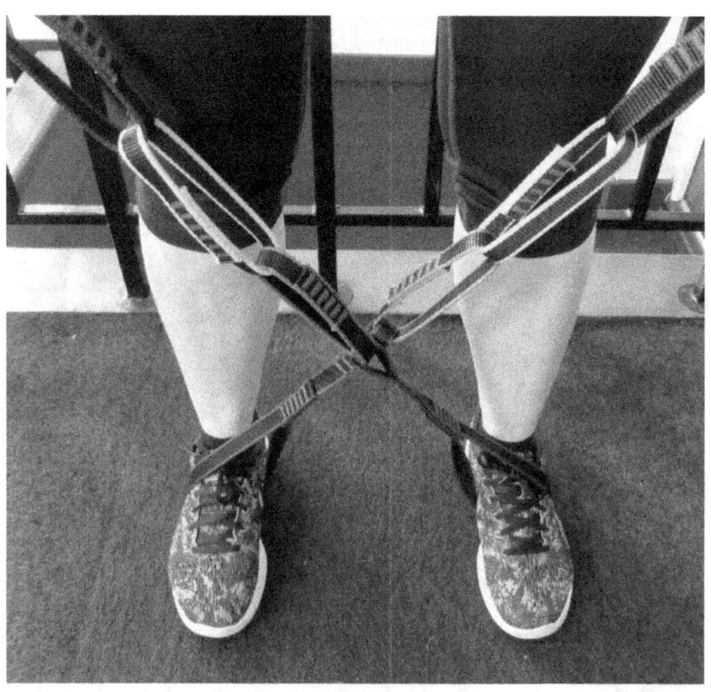

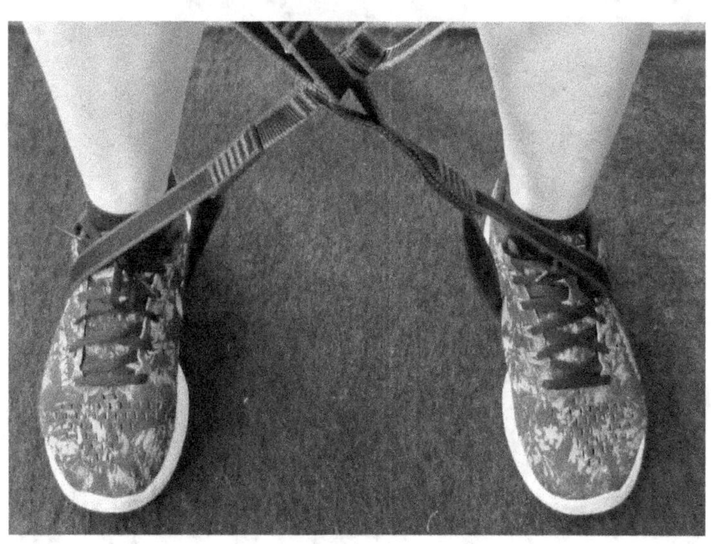

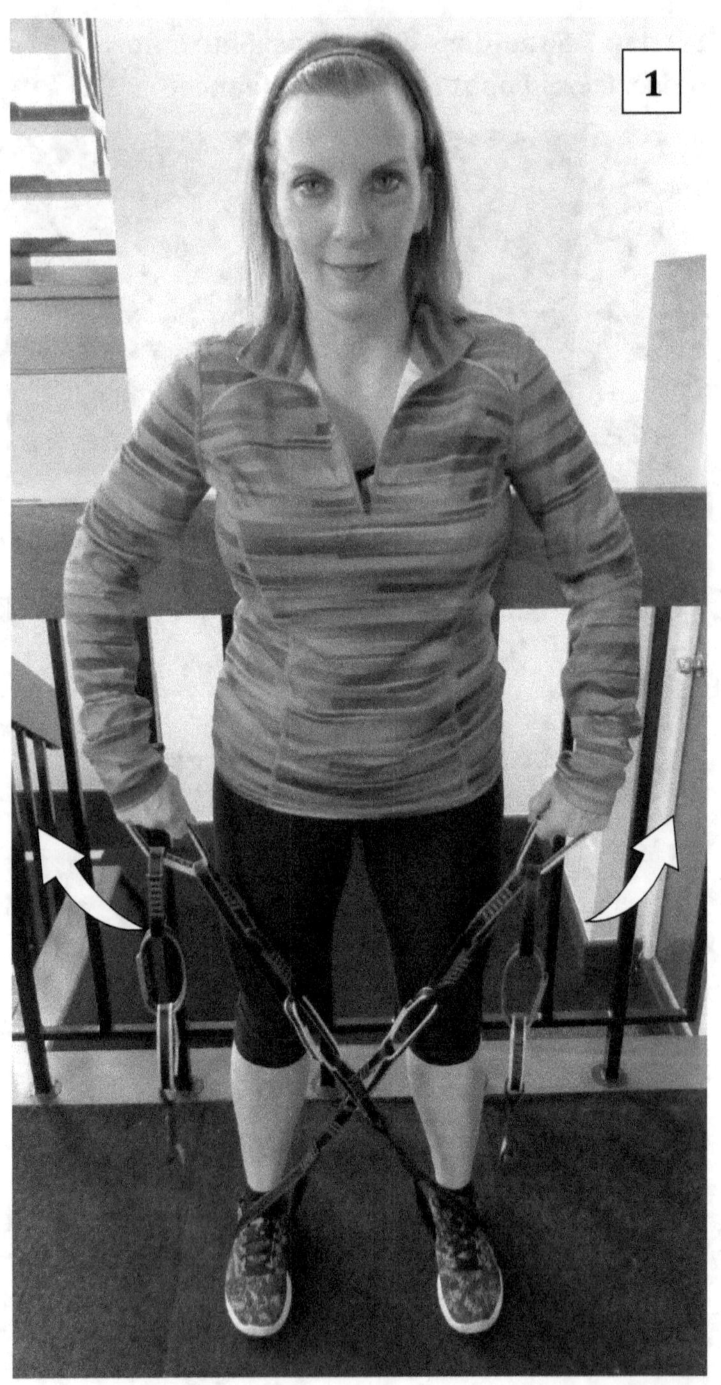

1

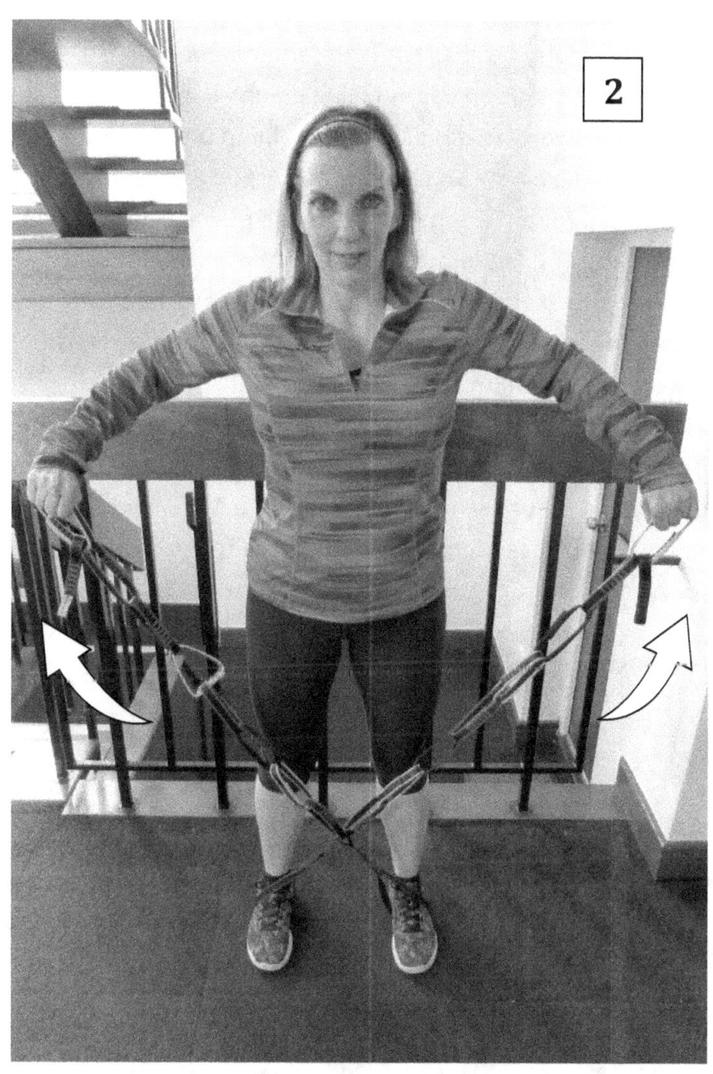

2

Section 7 Shoulders:

Front Raise

Stand upright and place your feet in each foot loop of the two daisy chains. For general shoulder exercise, grip the same colour loop palms facing down at approximately mid-chest level on each daisy chain. Bend both arms slightly at the elbow and keep them locked in that position. Attempt to raise the arms forward and upwards in an arcing move. Use your shoulder muscles as the driving force to perform the exercise. Advanced users may wish to use increasingly wider or shorter daisy chain loops to exercise the shoulders at different points on the ROM (Range of Motion) of the arms and shoulders. When you perform an isometric exercise, never hold your breath. Always breathe deeply and naturally, which will be about 10 full breaths at a rate of about 1 second per breath.   Perform each exercise for no less than 7 seconds and no longer than 10.

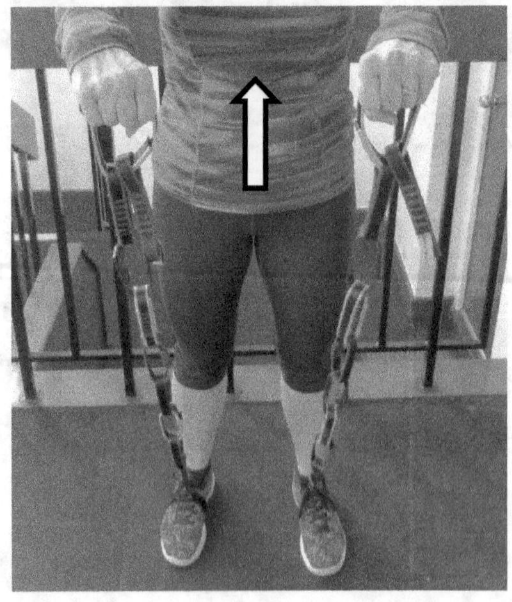

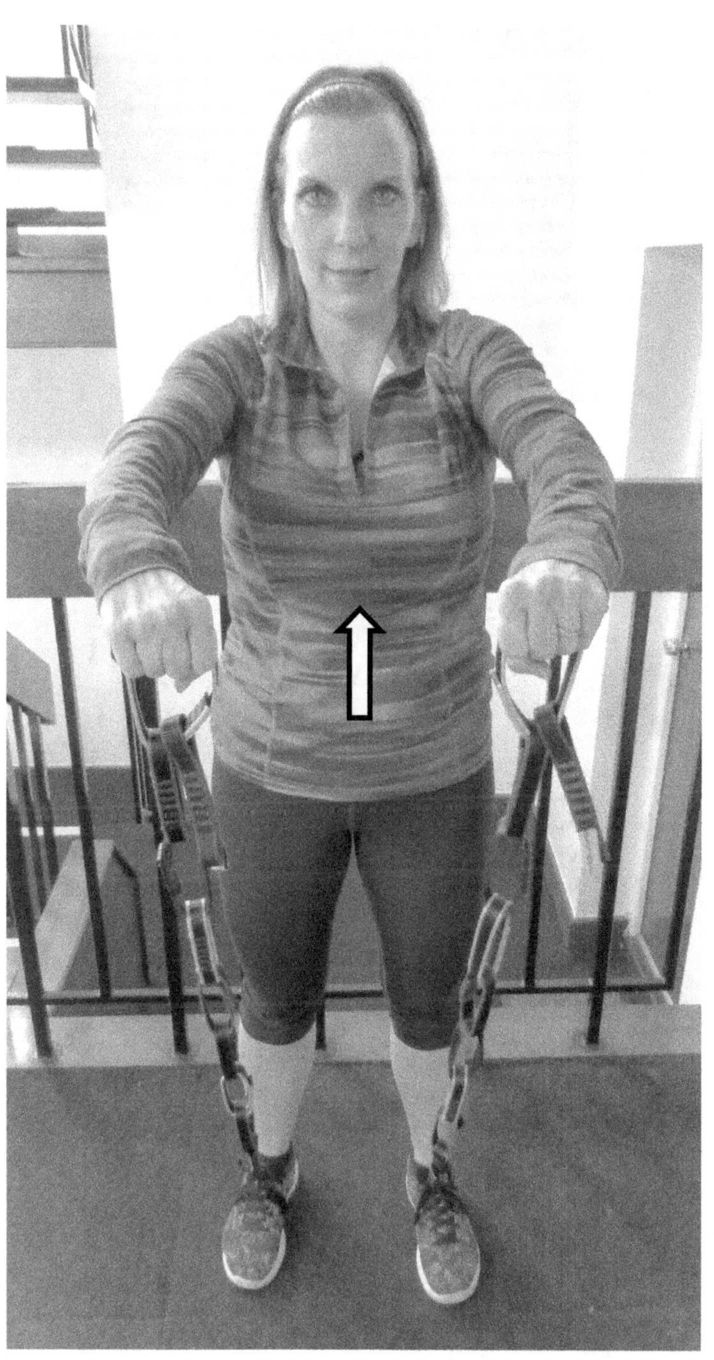

178

Section 7 Shoulders Variations:

Forward Raise – Wider Loops

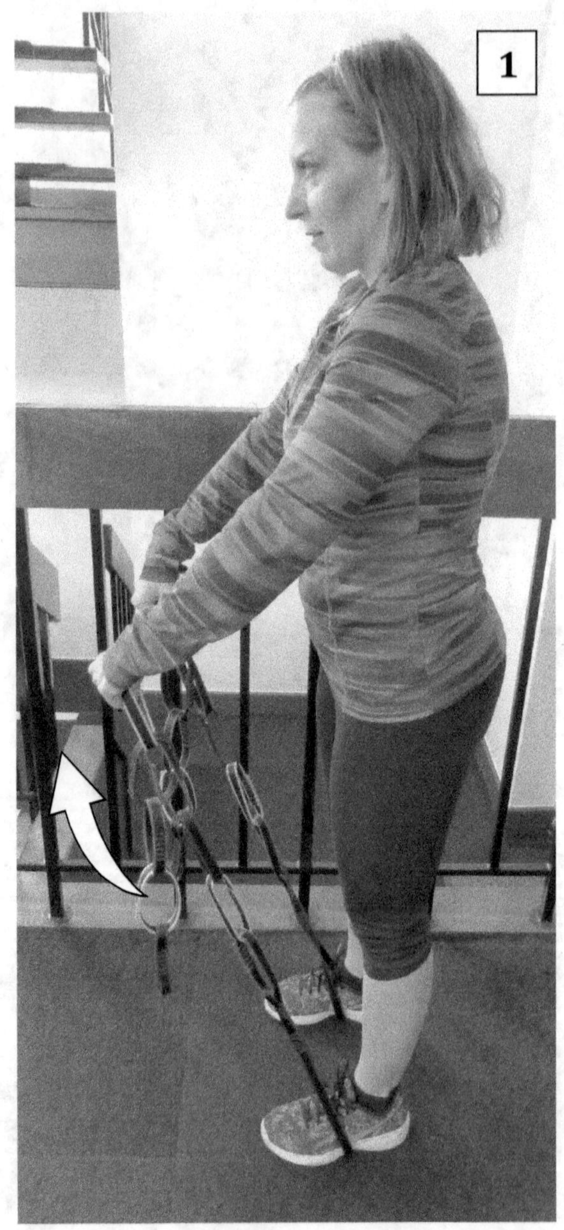

179

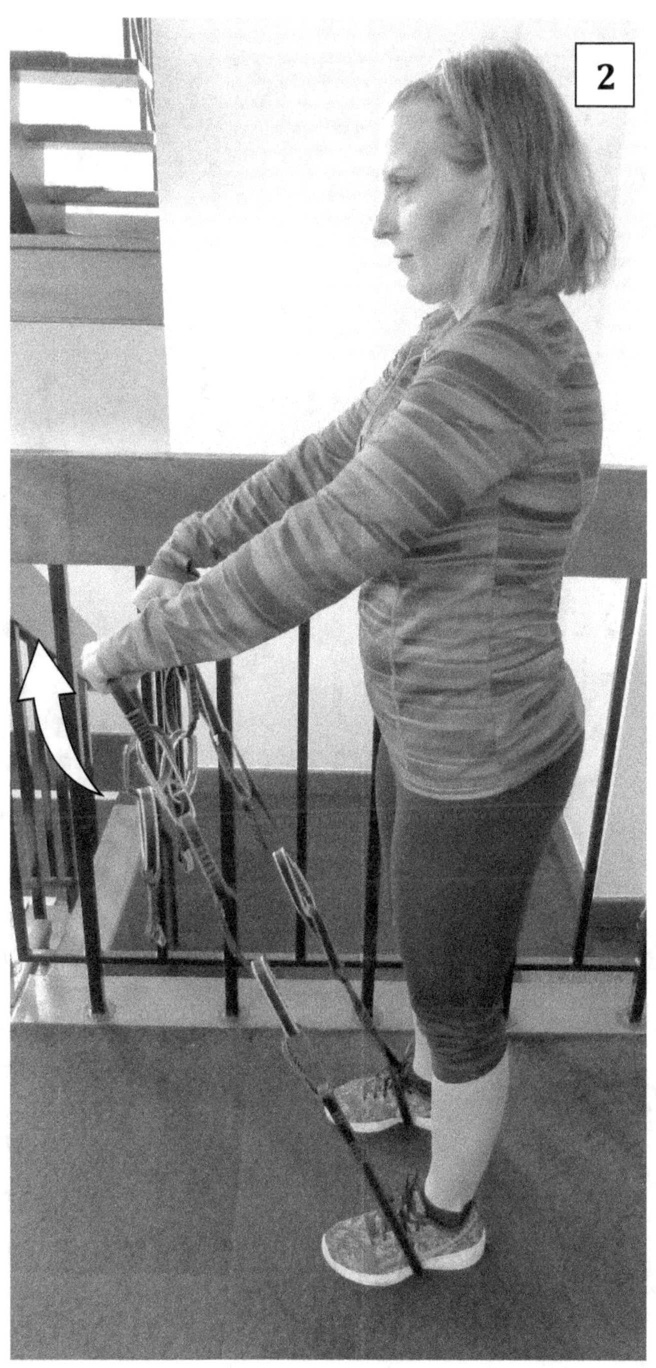

2

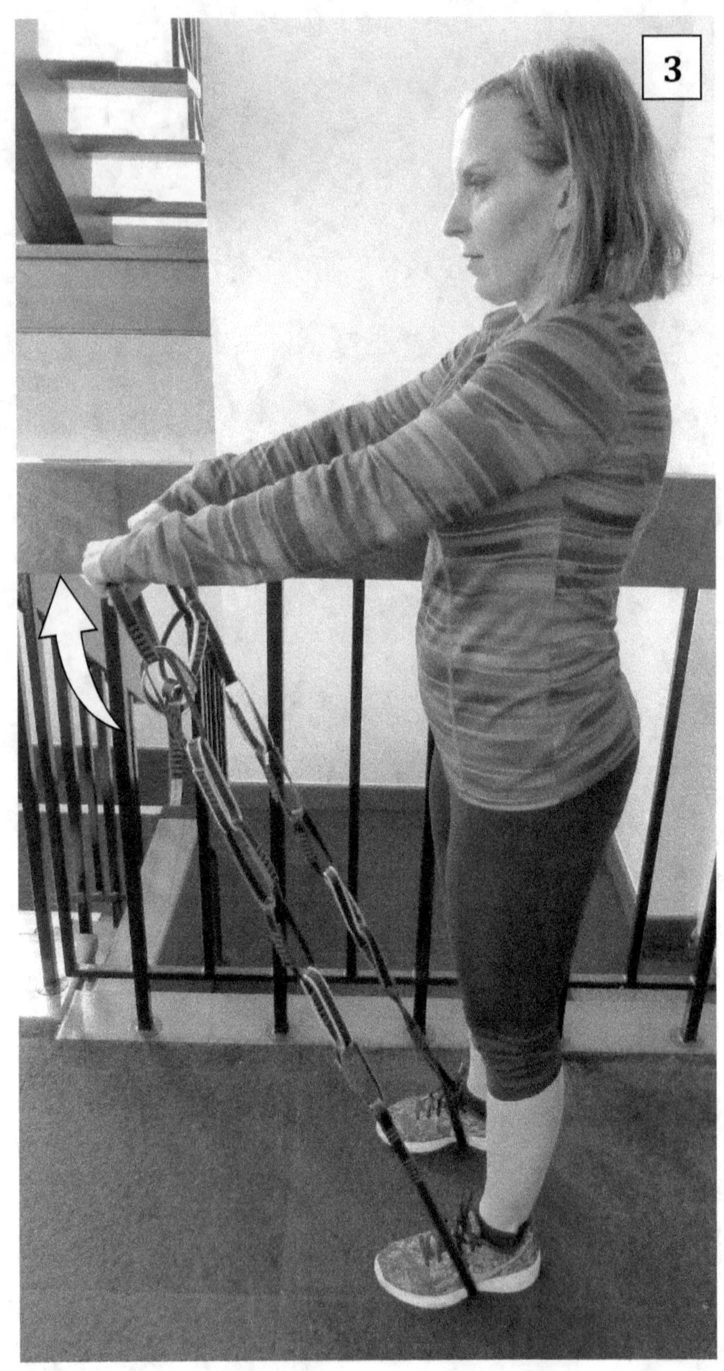
3

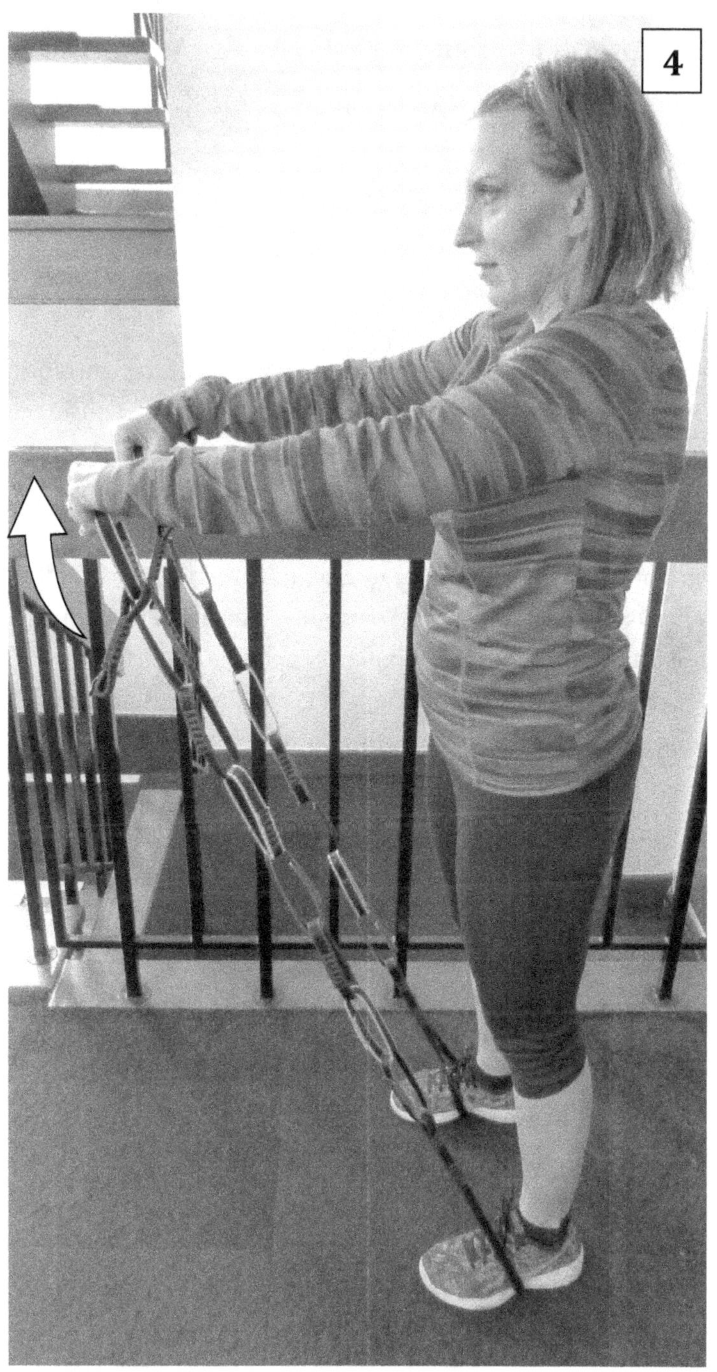

4

Section 7 Shoulders:

Single-Arm Standing Press

Connect two daisy chains with a carabiner. Stand upright and place your feet in a foot loop of one daisy chain. For general shoulder exercise, grip a mid-point loop with your palms facing forward on the upper daisy chain. Bend the arm at the elbow to approximately 90 degrees if possible. Align the body, hips and legs in a neutral position and then engage the shoulder and neck muscles to push upwards with the hand holding the loop. Advanced users may wish to use other loops to exercise the shoulder at different points on the ROM, or Range of Motion. When you perform an isometric exercise, never hold your breath. Always breathe deeply and naturally, which will be about 10 full breaths at a rate of about 1 second per breath. Perform each exercise for no less than 7 seconds and no longer than 10. Exercise both sides in the same way.

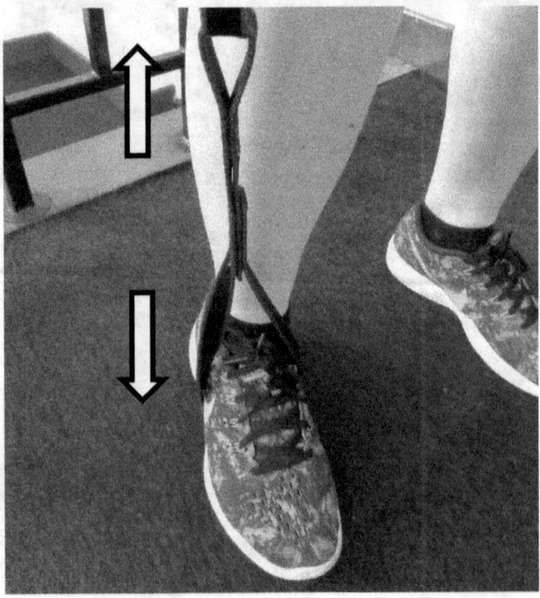

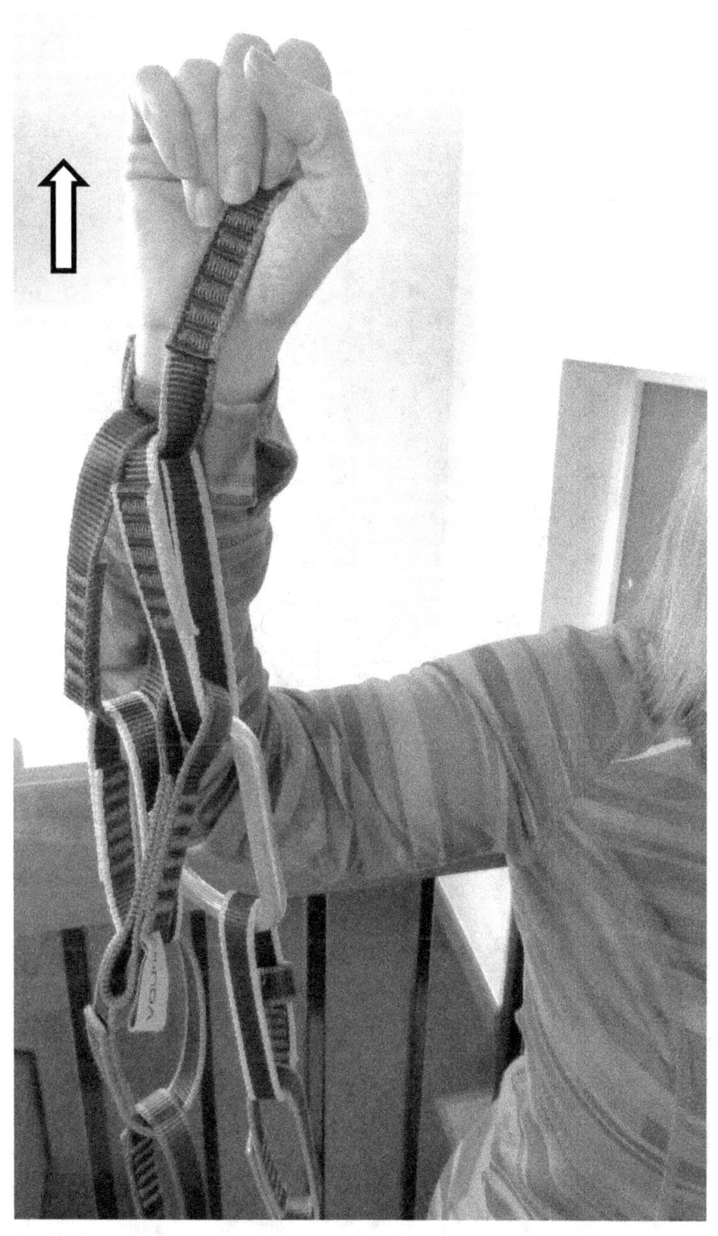

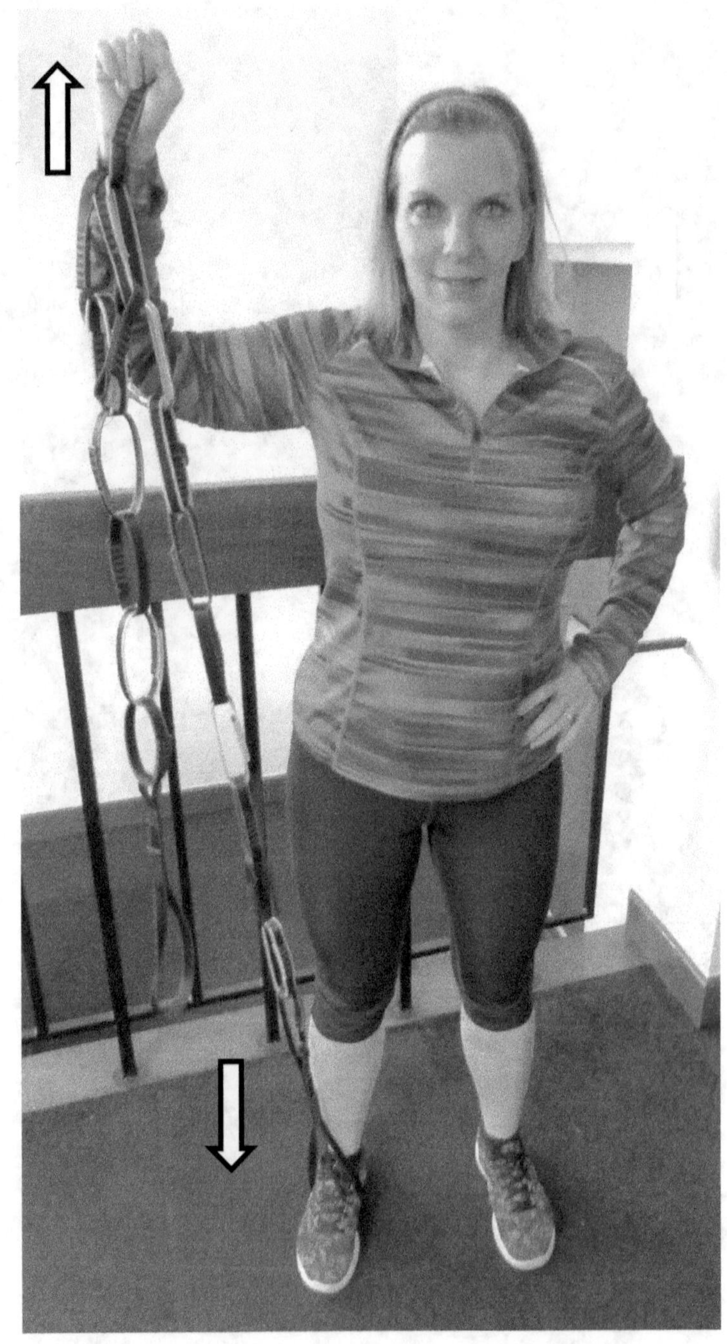

185

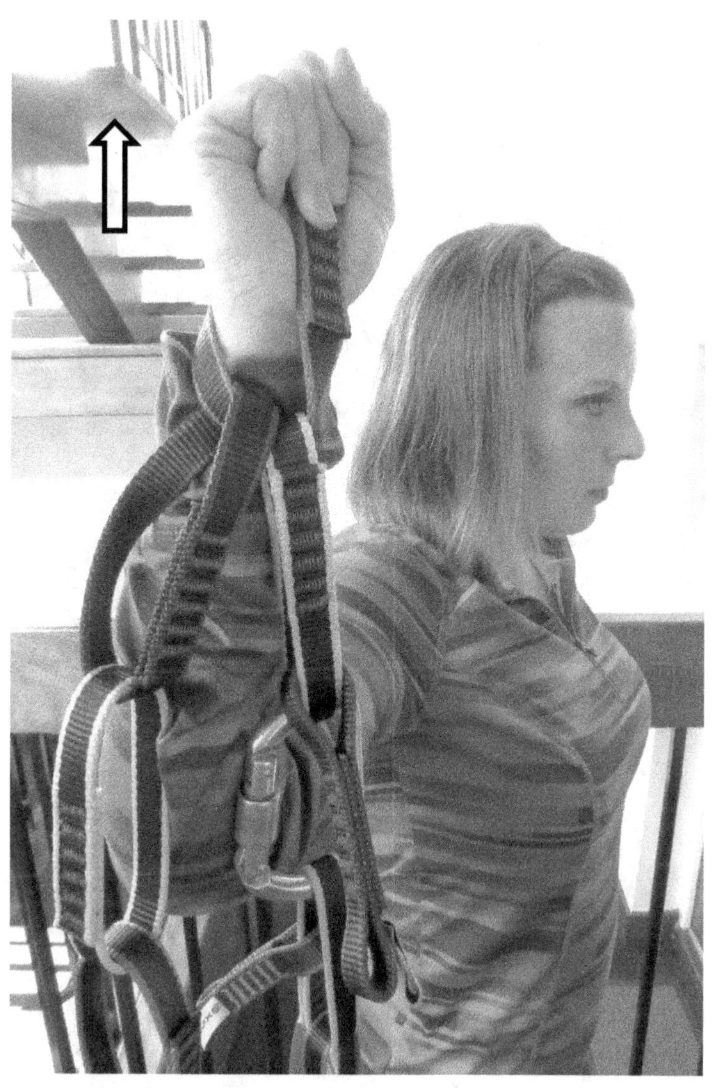

Section 7 Shoulders: Carabiner Linking

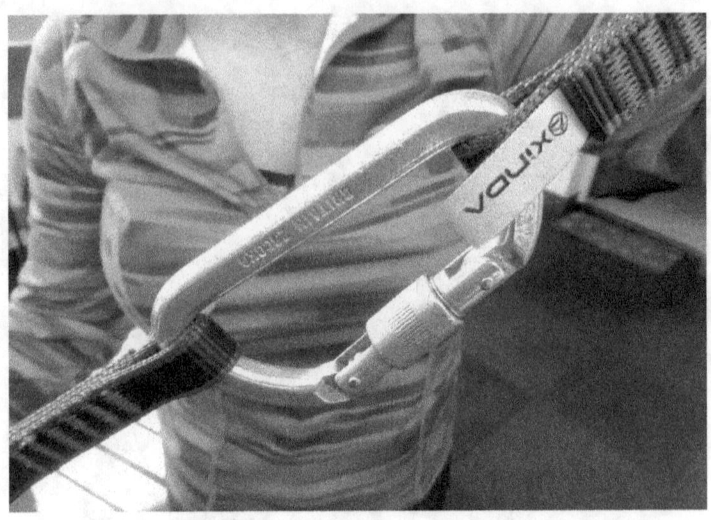

Extending a Daisy Chain Without a Carabiner by Adding a Looped Climbing Sling
<u>NOTE</u>: When Using a Climbing Sling, Use the Sling as a Foot Loop to Extend the Daisy Chain Higher

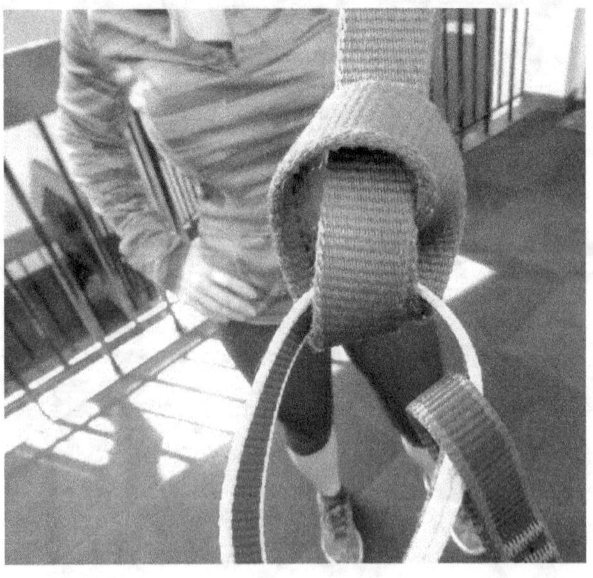

Extended Daisy Chain with Climbing Sling

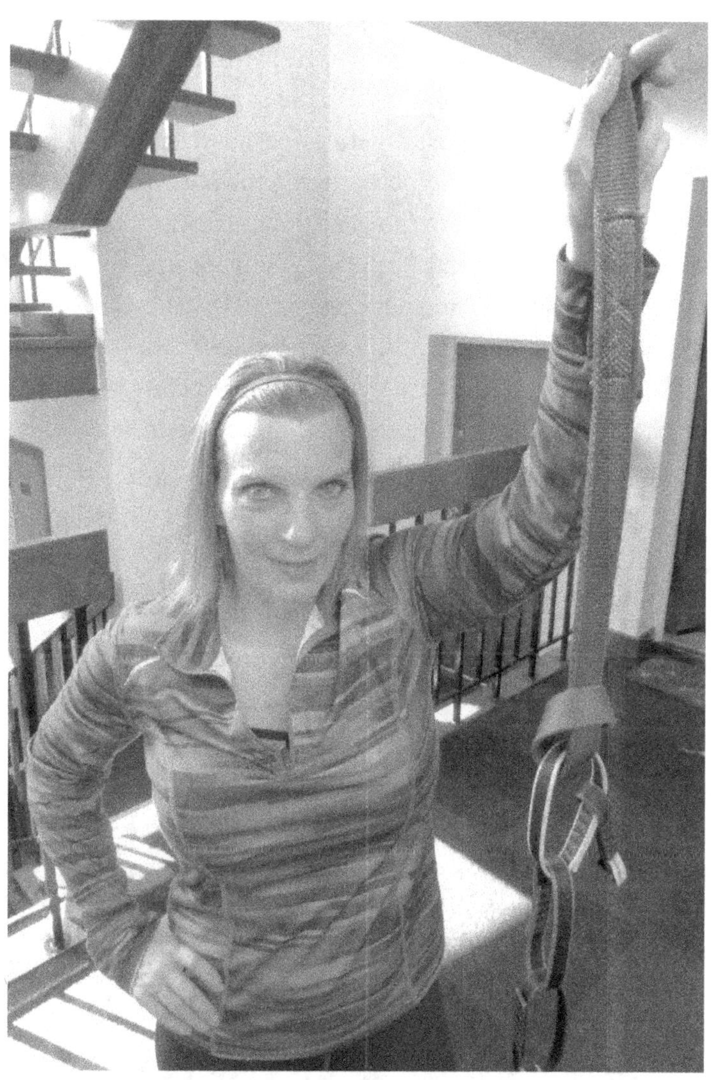

Section 7 Shoulders:

Upright Row

Stand upright and place one foot in each foot loop of two daisy chains. Hold both arms in front of you at waist height. For general exercise, grip the same colour loop of each daisy chain at approximately mid-point between your hips and chest with your palms facing towards you. Keep your arms slightly twisted to keep your elbows forward. Align the body, hips and legs in a neutral position and then engage the shoulder and neck muscles to pull upwards with the hands holding the loops. Advanced users may wish to use other loops to exercise the shoulder at different points on the ROM - Range of Motion. When you perform an isometric exercise, never hold your breath. Always breathe deeply and naturally, which will be about 10 full breaths at a rate of about 1 second per breath.   Perform each exercise for no less than 7 seconds and no longer than 10.

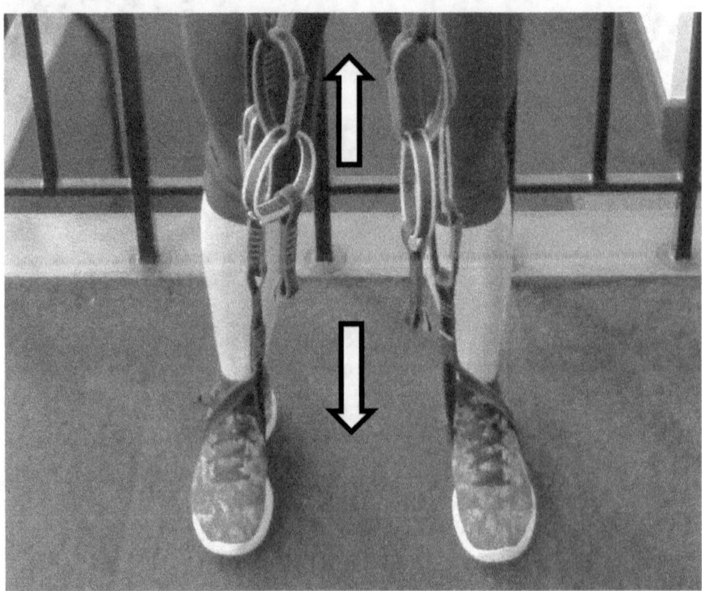

1

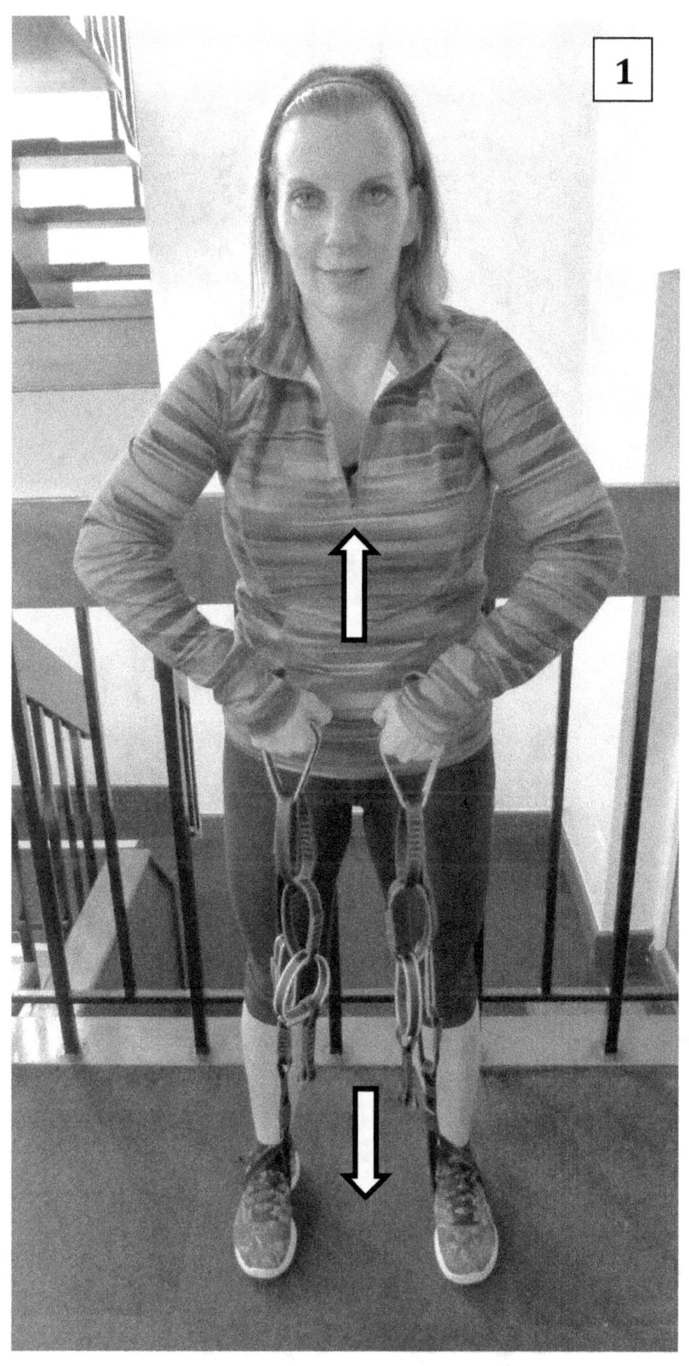

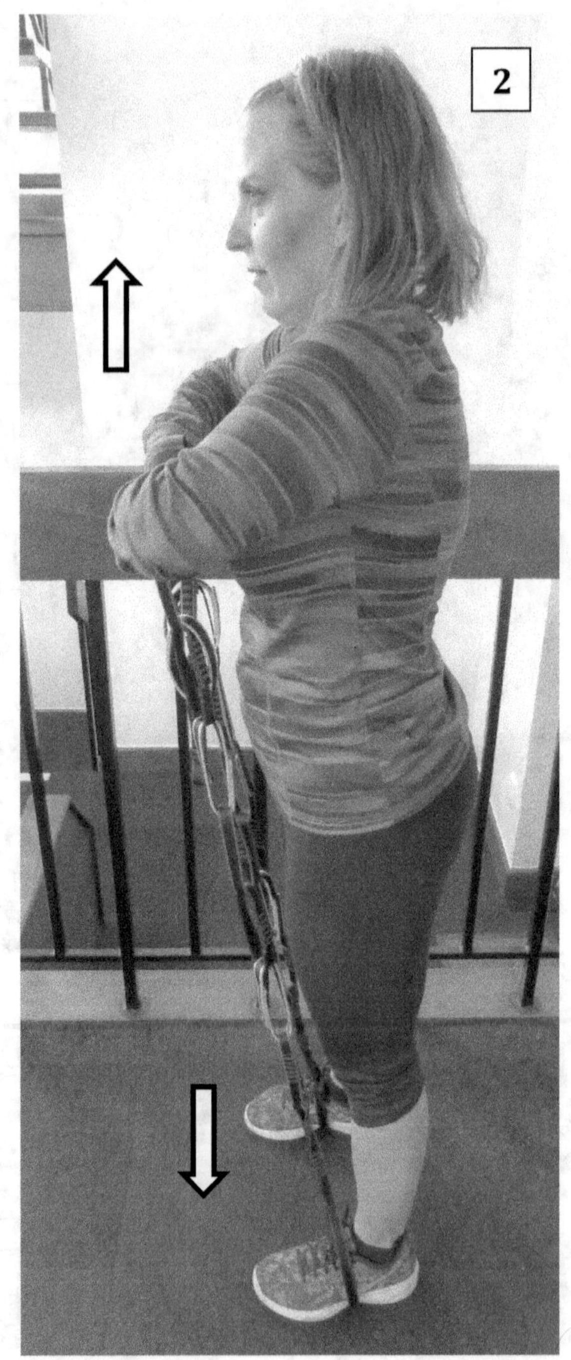

2

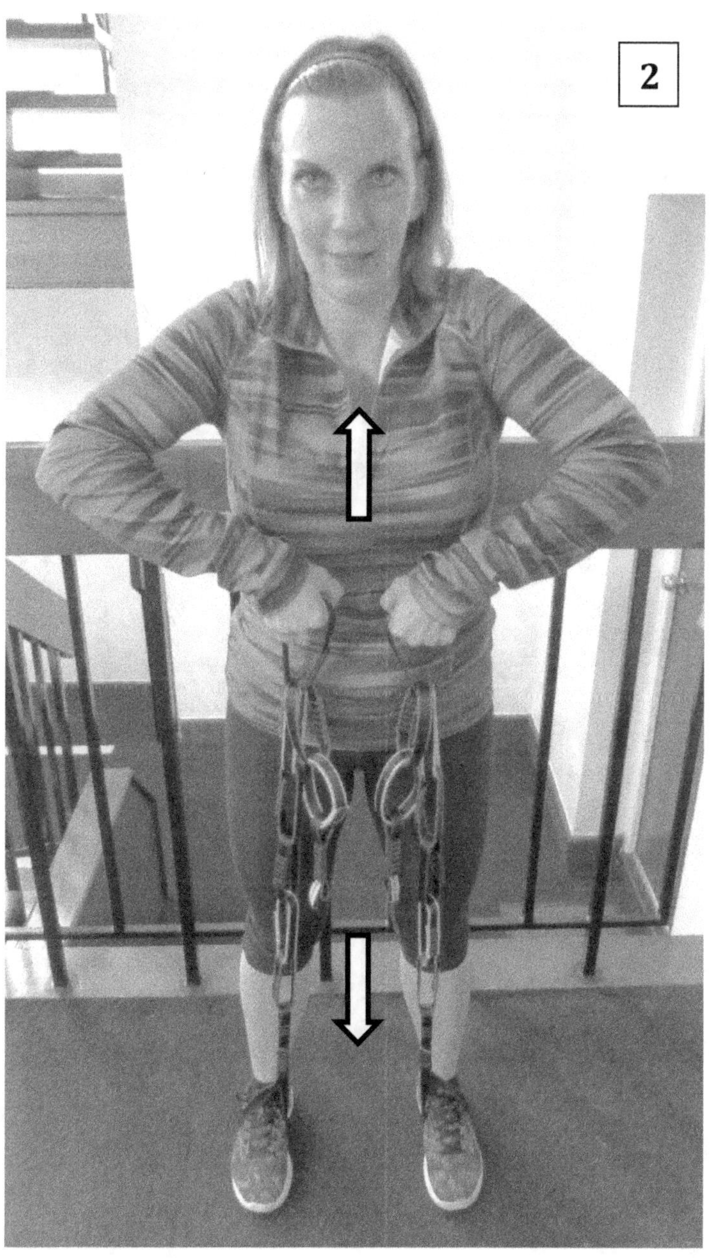

2

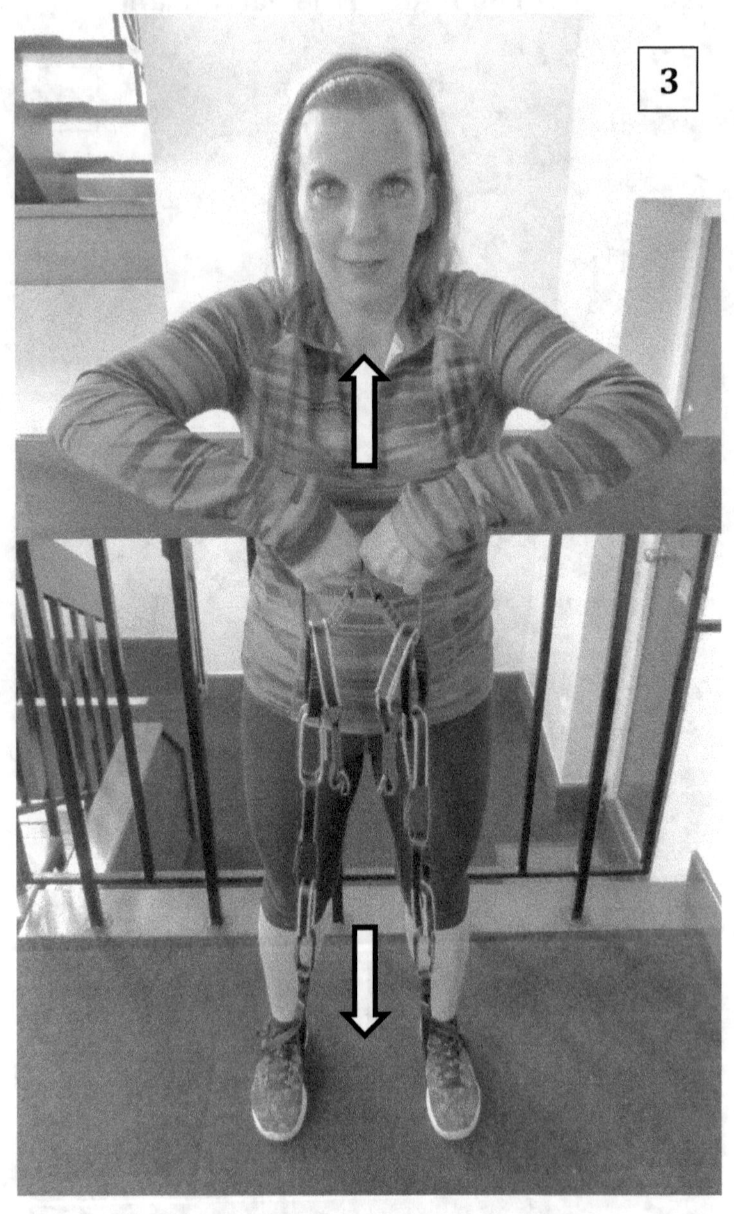

3

Section 8 Thighs Front:

Wall Squat and Leg Press

Although this exercise is not necessarily one that uses a daisy chain, it is an excellent front-thigh exercise, which is why we have included it. Stand with your feet about shoulder-width apart, slightly away from a solid wall or object. Squat down while leaning against the object with your entire torso and glutes. Pushing backwards and slightly upwards, attempt to stand up from the lower squat position to engage the thighs and glutes to perform the exercise. Advanced users would exercise at different positions/angles of squat depth. When you perform an isometric exercise, never hold your breath. Always breathe deeply and naturally, which will be about 10 full breaths at a rate of about 1 second per breath. Perform each exercise for no less than 7 seconds and no longer than 10.

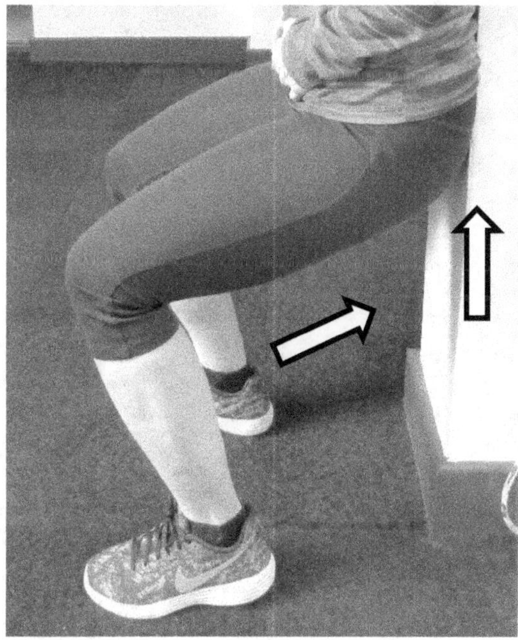

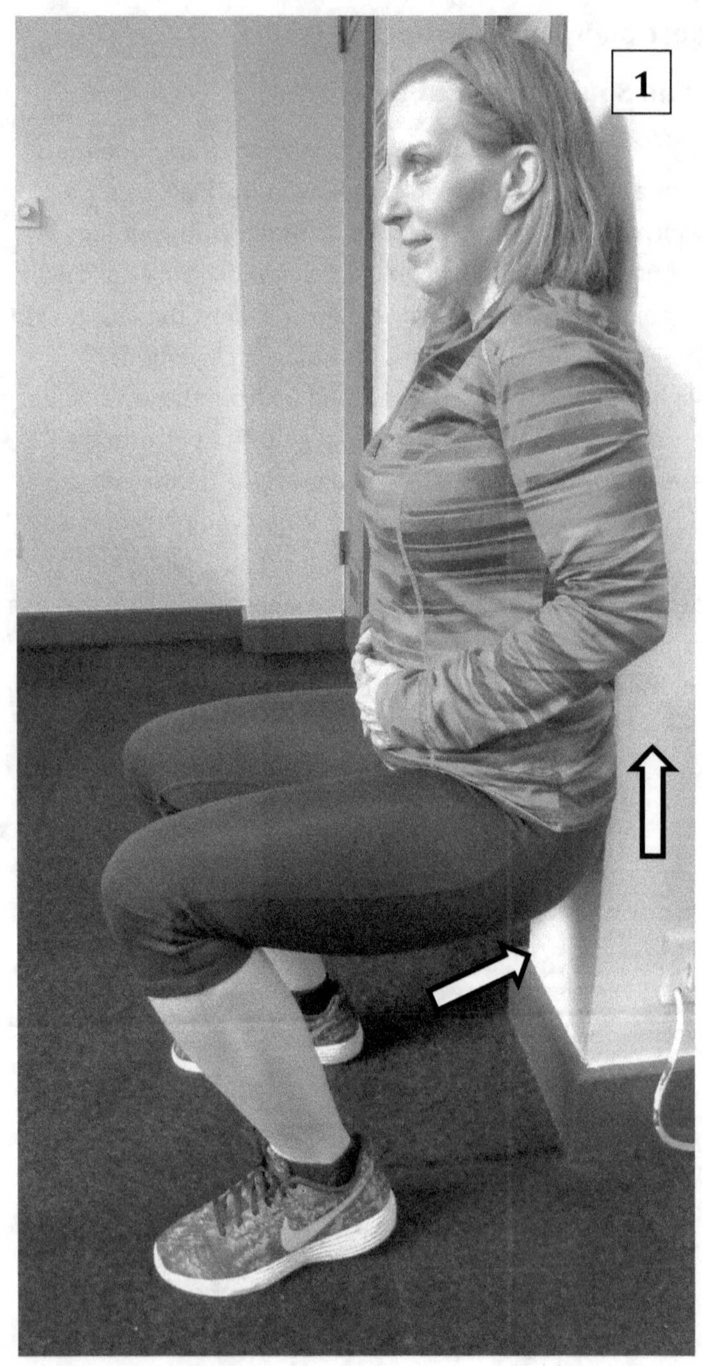

1

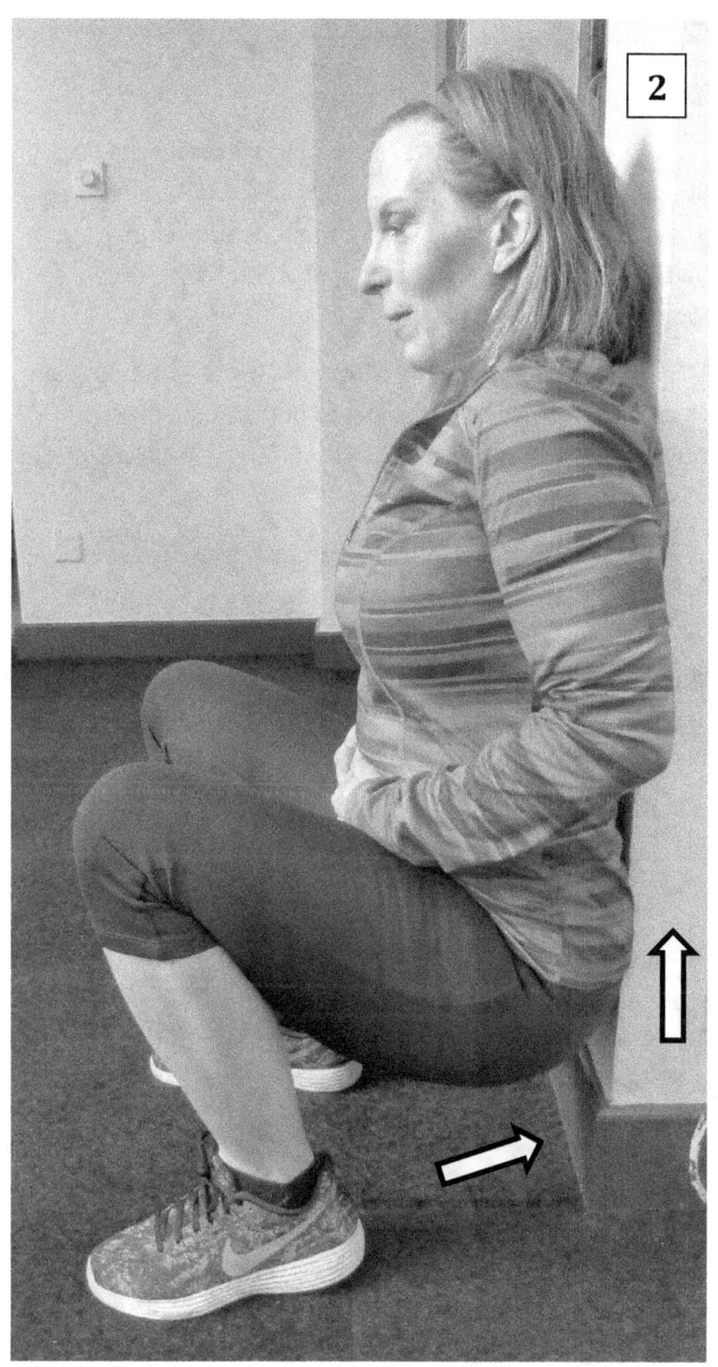
2

Section 8 Thighs Front:

The Squat

Place one foot in each loop of two daisy chains. Stand with your feet approximately shoulder-width apart. Squat down, bending only from the hips and keeping your back straight. Take hold of an appropriate same-coloured loop on each daisy chain.

Attempt to stand up from the lower squat position to engage the thighs and glutes to perform the exercise. Advanced users would exercise at different positions/angles of squat depth.

When you perform an isometric exercise, never hold your breath. Always breathe deeply and naturally, which will be about 10 full breaths at a rate of about 1 second per breath. Perform each exercise for no less than 7 seconds and no longer than 10.

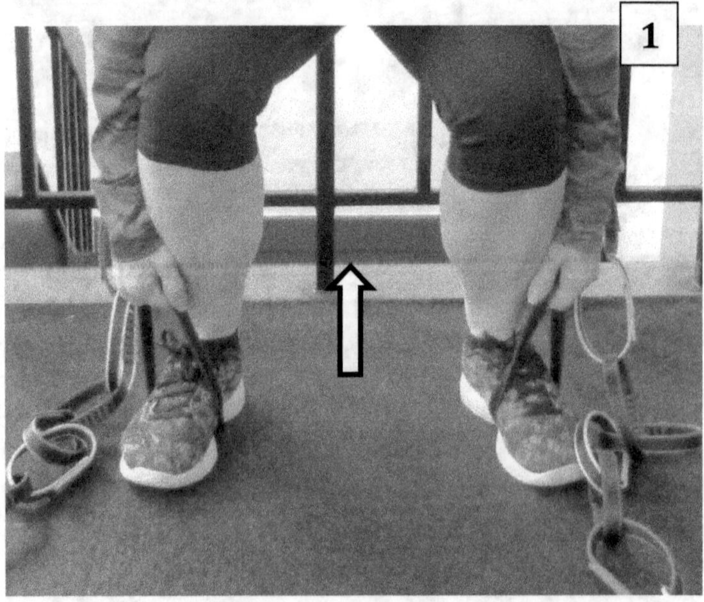

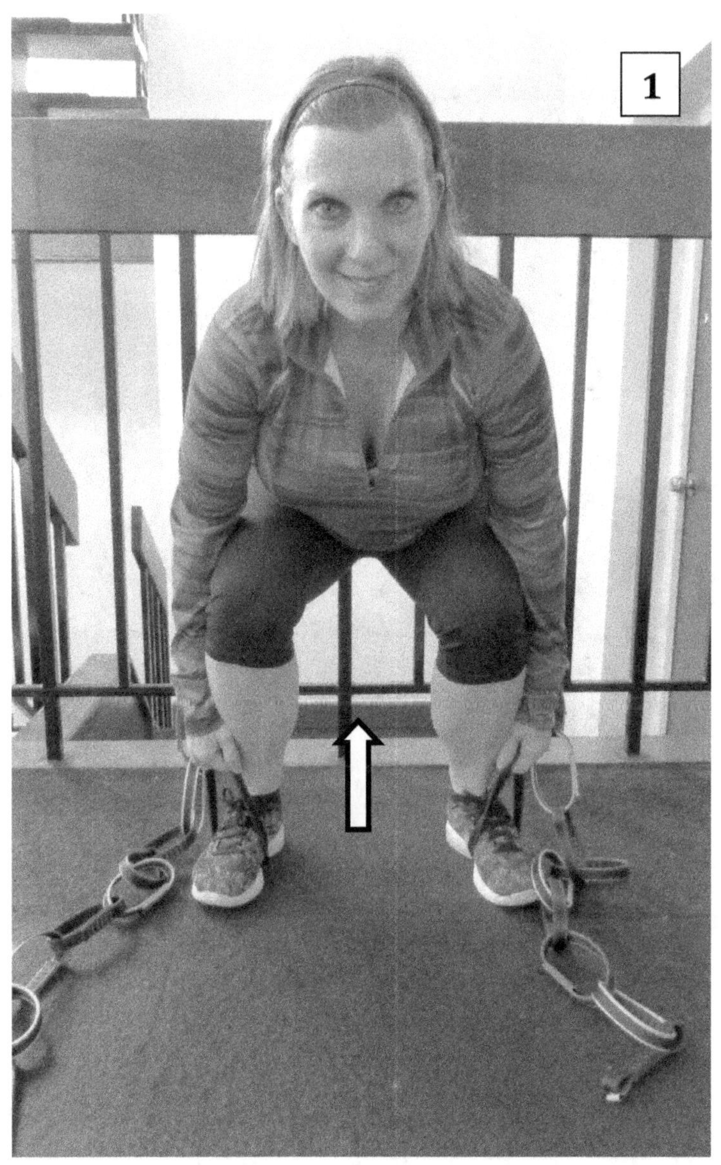

1

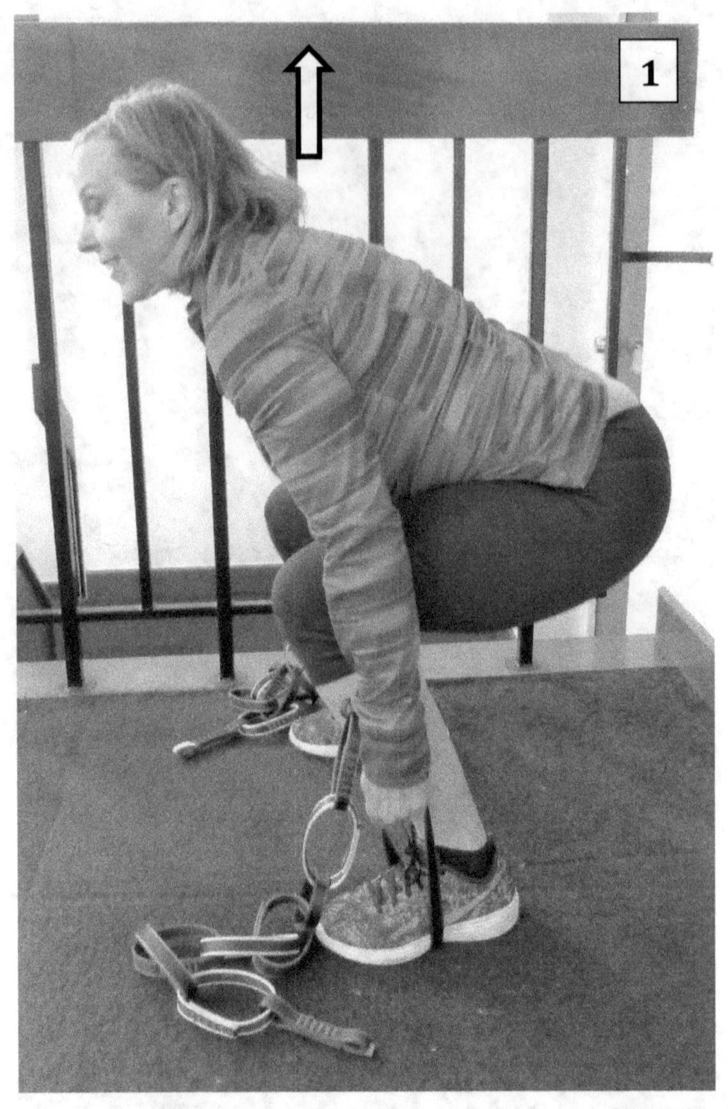

199

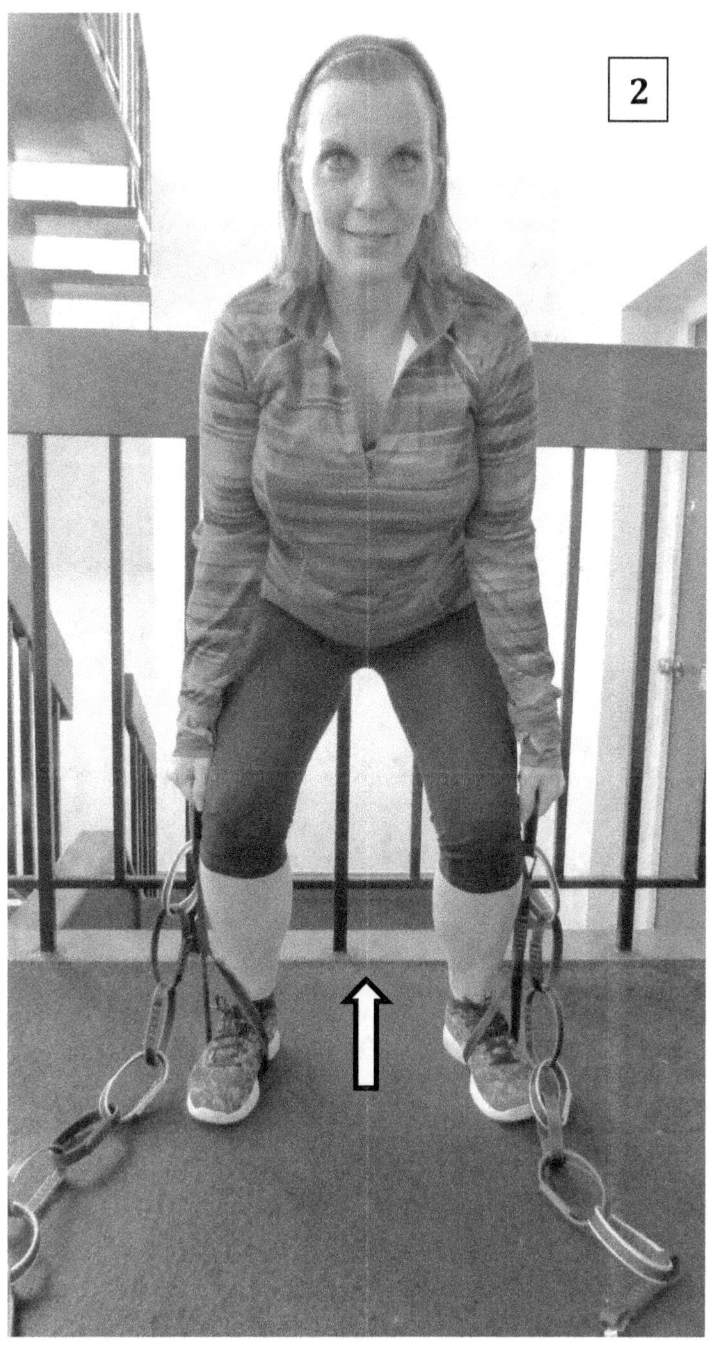

2

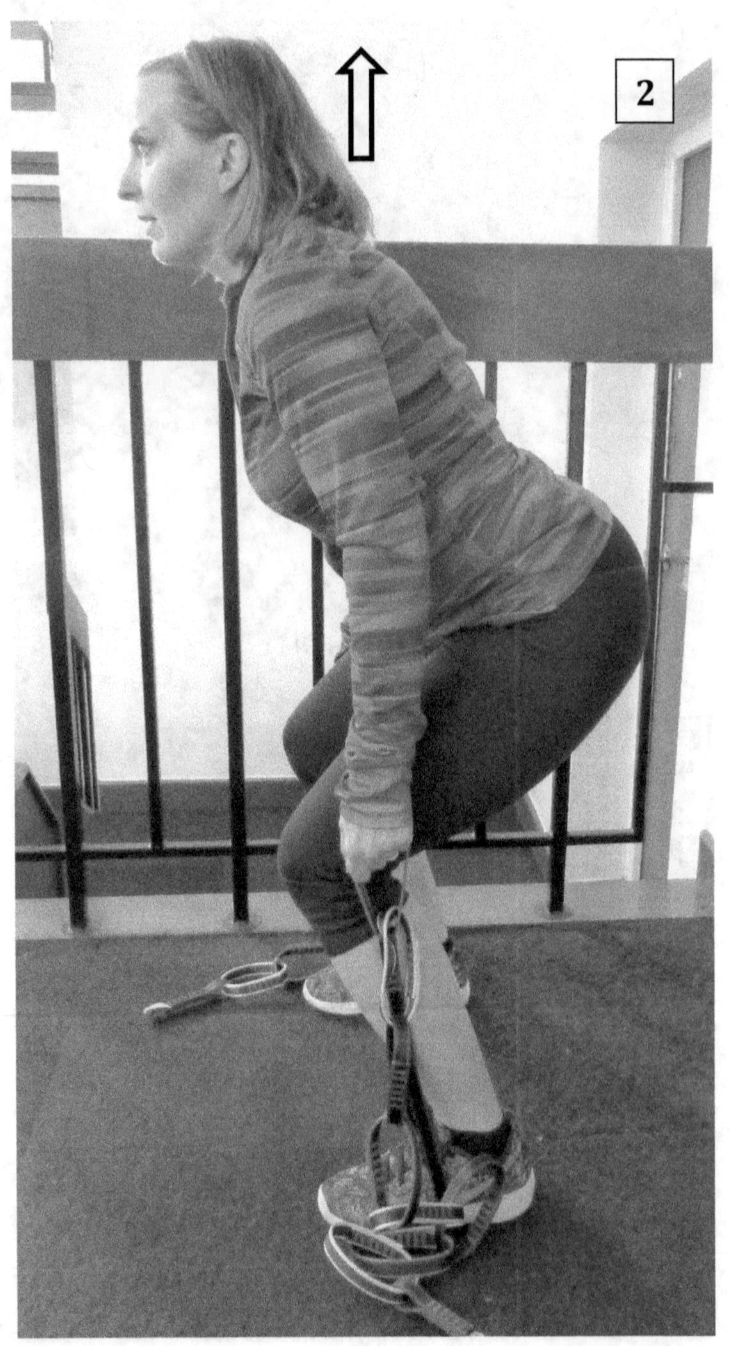

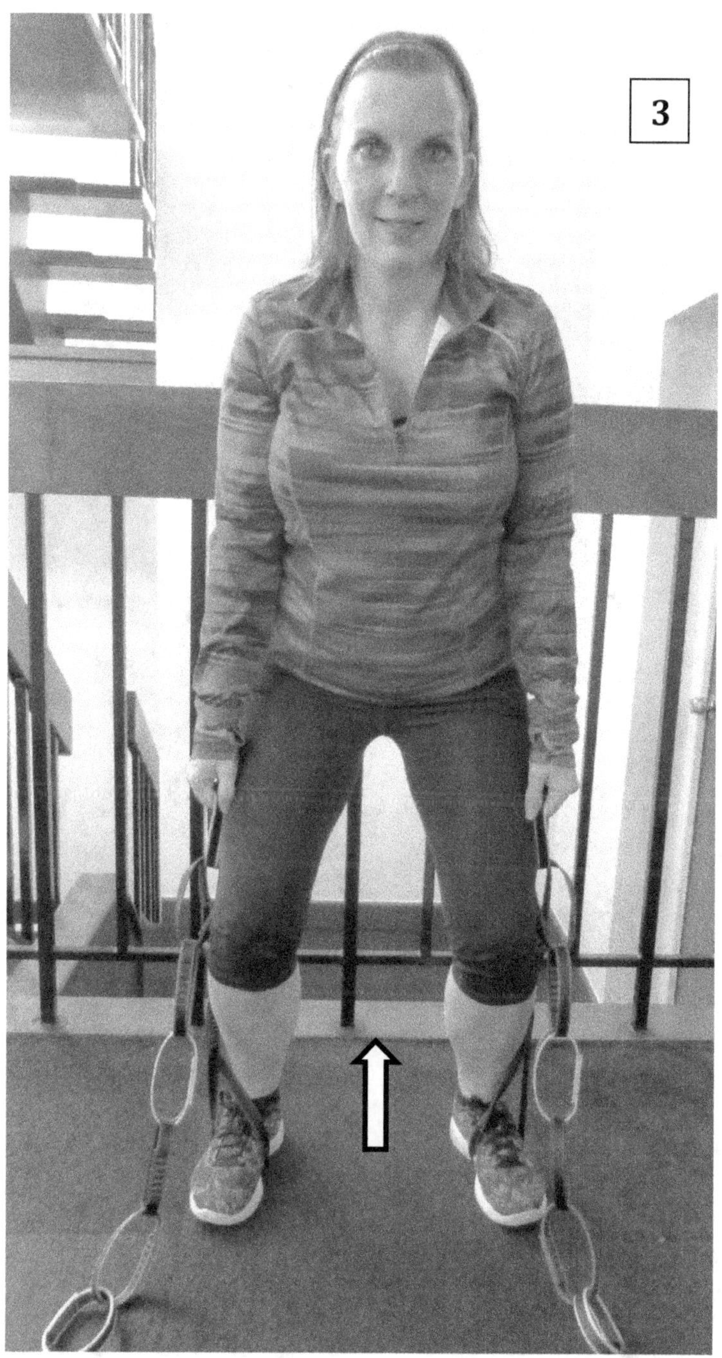

3

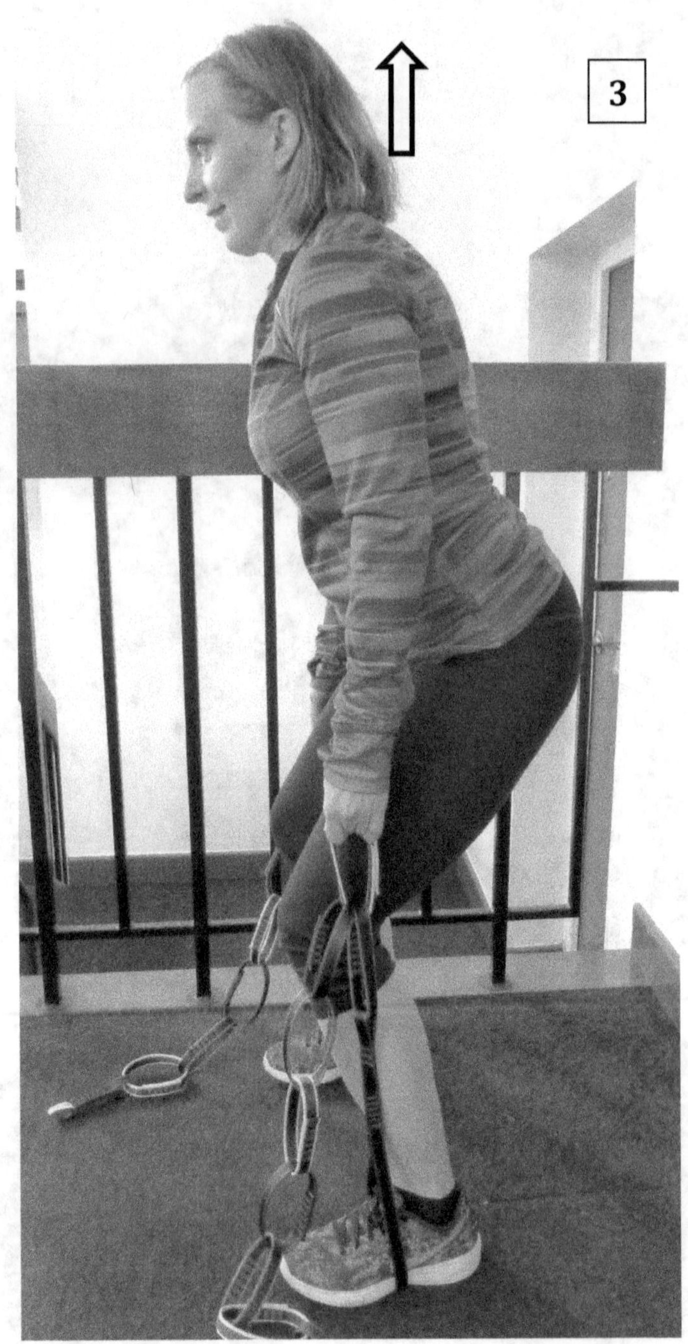

3

Section 8 Thighs Front:

Forward Split Squat

Stand upright with your feet about shoulder-width apart. First: Step one pace forward with one foot and squat down into a split squat position. Place the same foot in each loop of two daisy chains. Grip the same colour loop on each daisy chain. Keep your torso and head as upright as possible. Attempt to return to an upright position from the lower split squat position by engaging the thighs and glutes to perform the exercise. Advanced variations would be at several different depth positions of the split squat along the ROM, or Range of Motion. When you perform an isometric exercise, never hold your breath. Always breathe deeply and naturally, which will be about 10 full breaths at a rate of about 1 second per breath. Perform each exercise for no less than 7 seconds and no longer than 10.

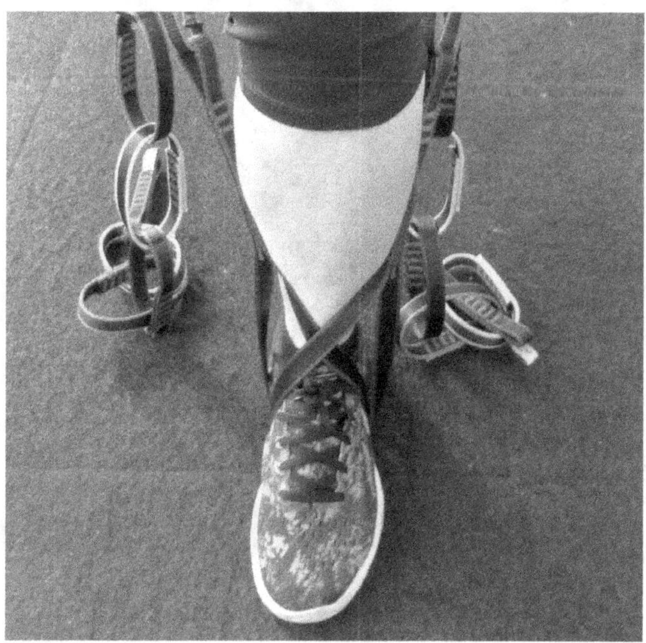

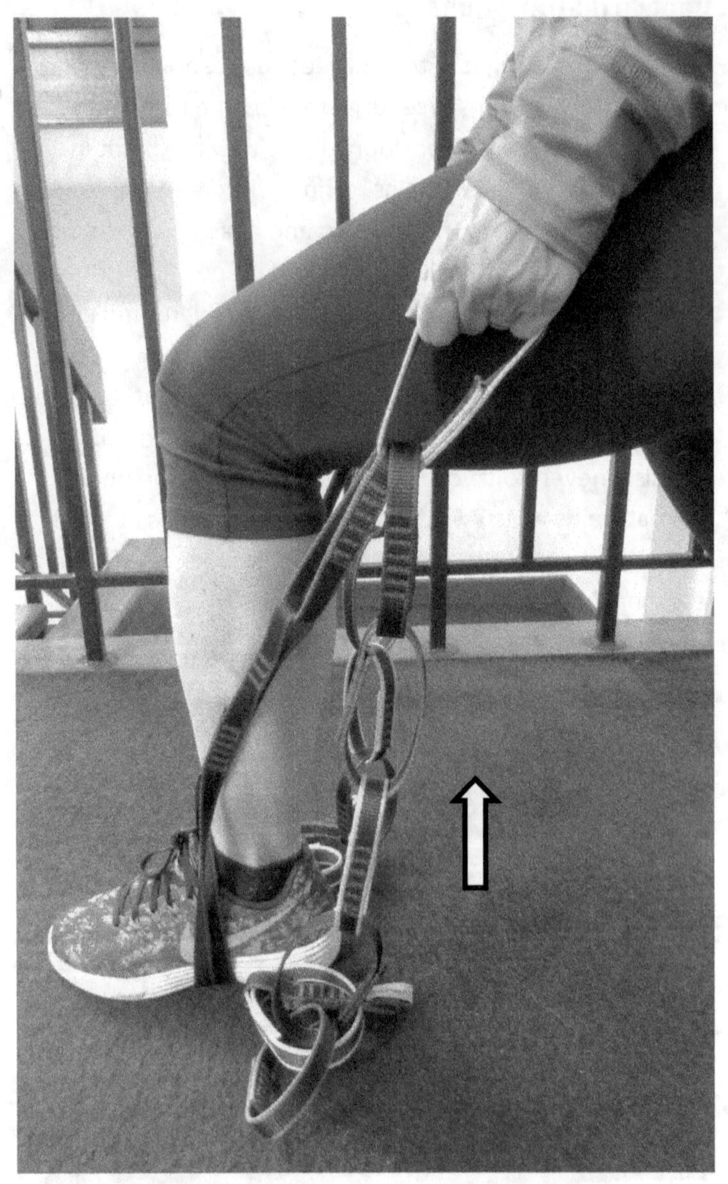

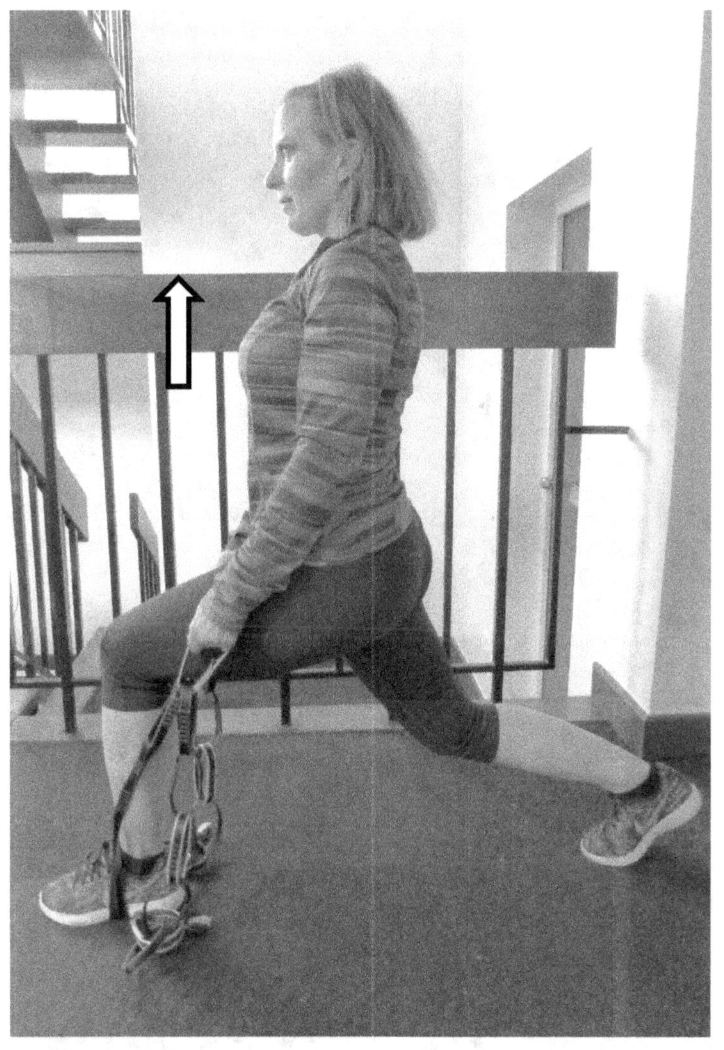

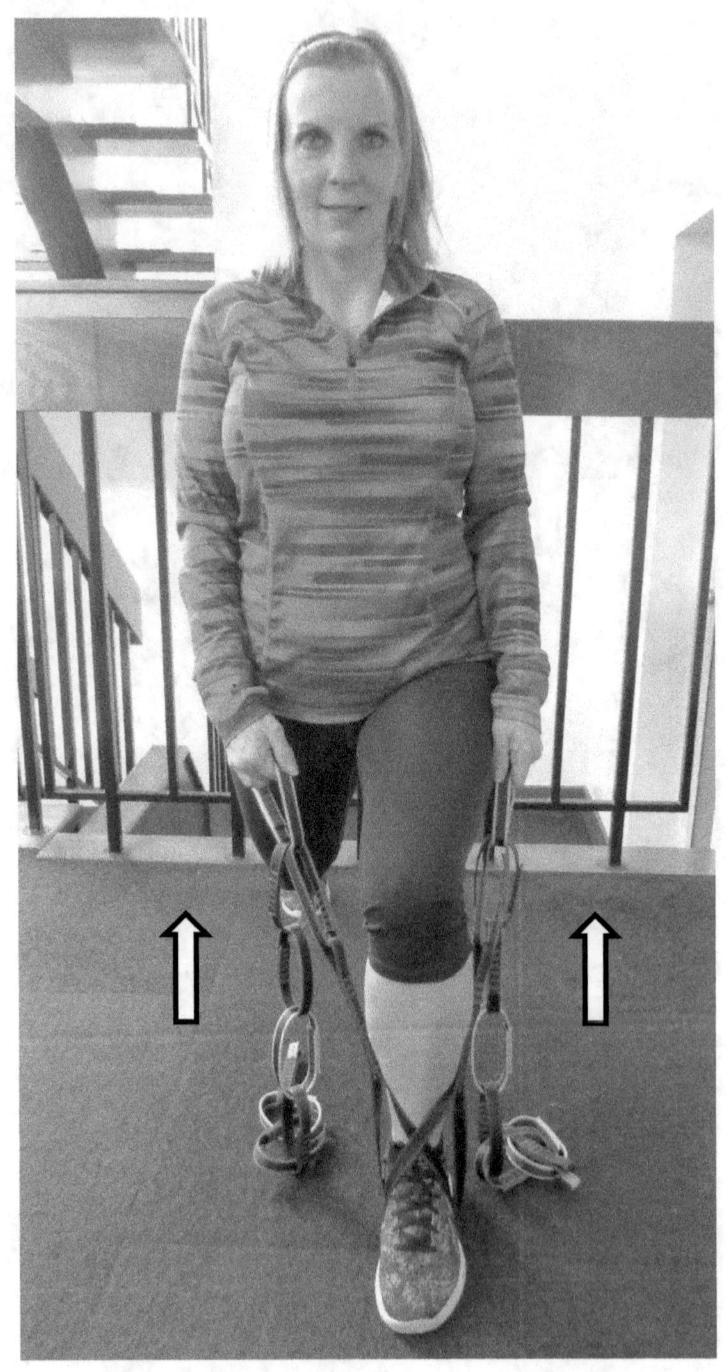

Section 8 Thighs Front:

Leg Extension

Sit on a bench or stool and raise one leg and knee in front of you with your foot close to the stool. Place the foot in the foot loop of two daisy chains. Grip the same colour loop on each daisy chain. Using the front thigh muscles, attempt to extend and straighten the lower leg forwards. When you have reached the desired angle and level of applied force, perform the exercise. Advanced variations would be when the lower leg is exercised at different positions on the ROM, or Range of Motion.

When you perform an isometric exercise, never hold your breath. Always breathe deeply and naturally, which will be about 10 full breaths at a rate of about 1 second per breath. Perform each exercise for no less than 7 seconds and no longer than 10.

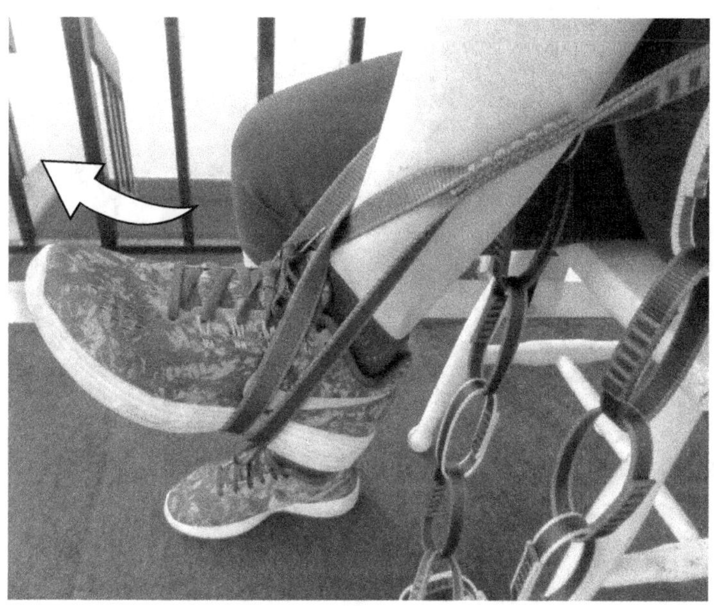

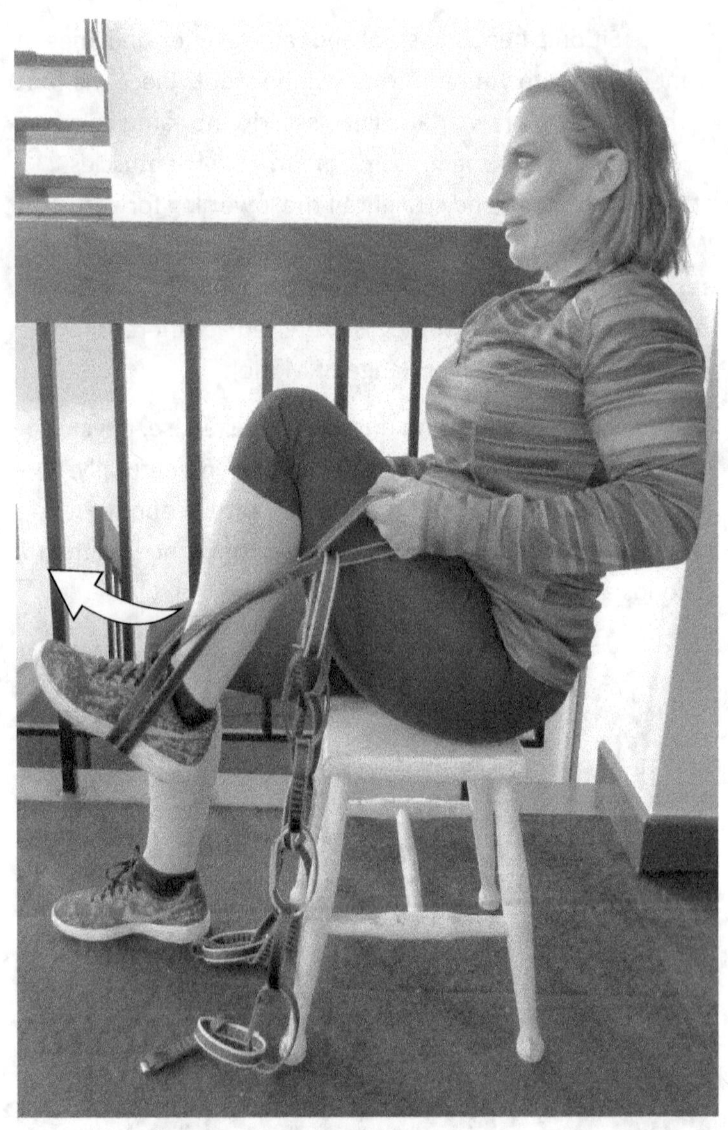

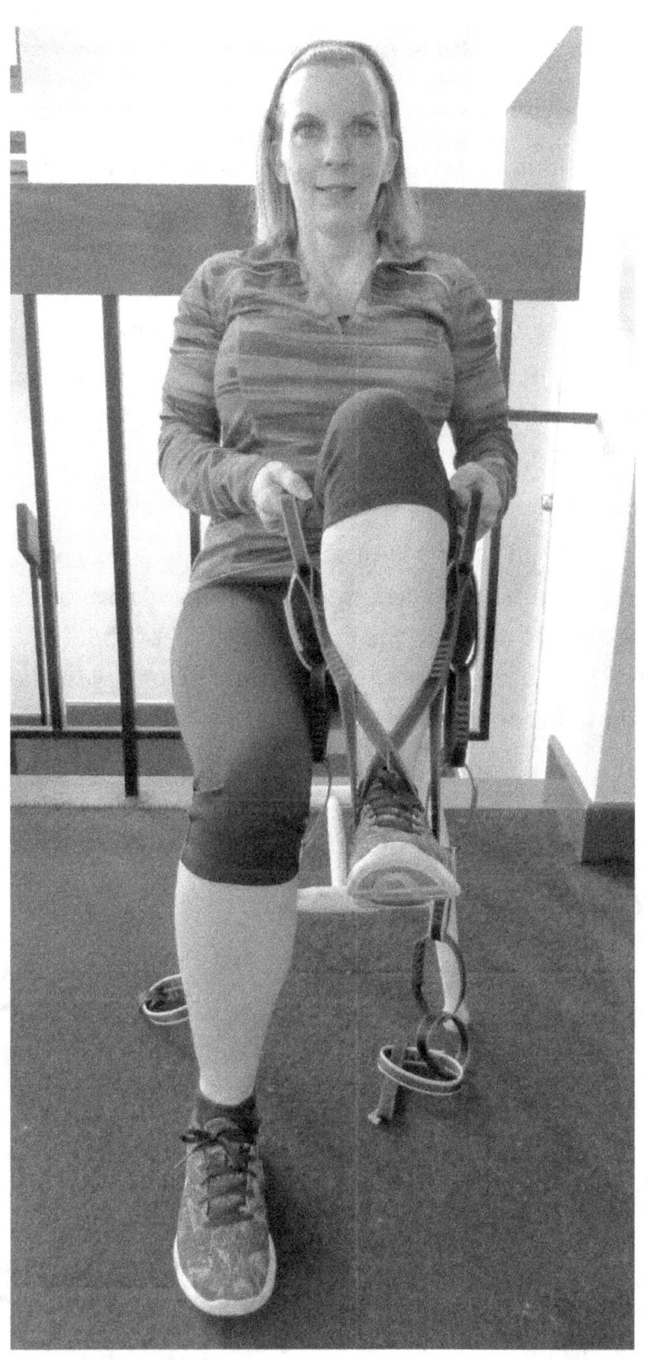

Section 8 Thighs Front and Side:

The Abductor

Sit on a bench or stool with your legs, knees, and feet together. Place a daisy chain over the lower thighs and grip a loop on each side. Use the outer thigh muscles to attempt to open the legs. This is prevented by pressing downwards with the daisy chain to resist any movement. When you have reached the desired angle and level of applied force, perform the exercise. Advanced variations would be when the exercise is performed at different positions on the ROM, or Range of Motion.

When you perform an isometric exercise, never hold your breath. Always breathe deeply and naturally, which will be about 10 full breaths at a rate of about 1 second per breath. Perform each exercise for no less than 7 seconds and no longer than 10.

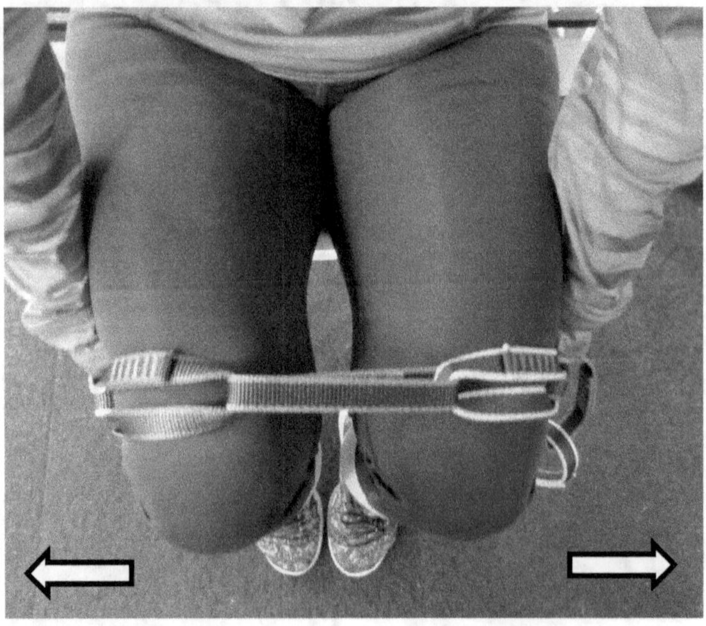

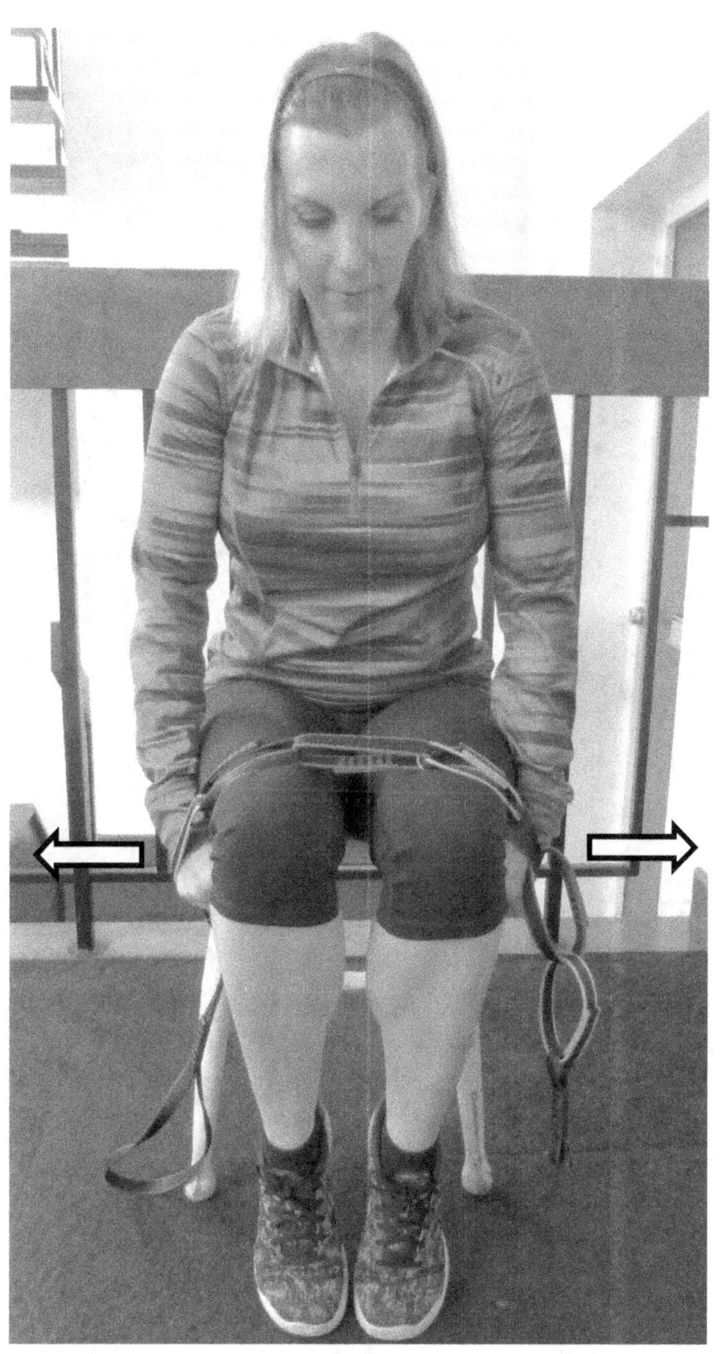

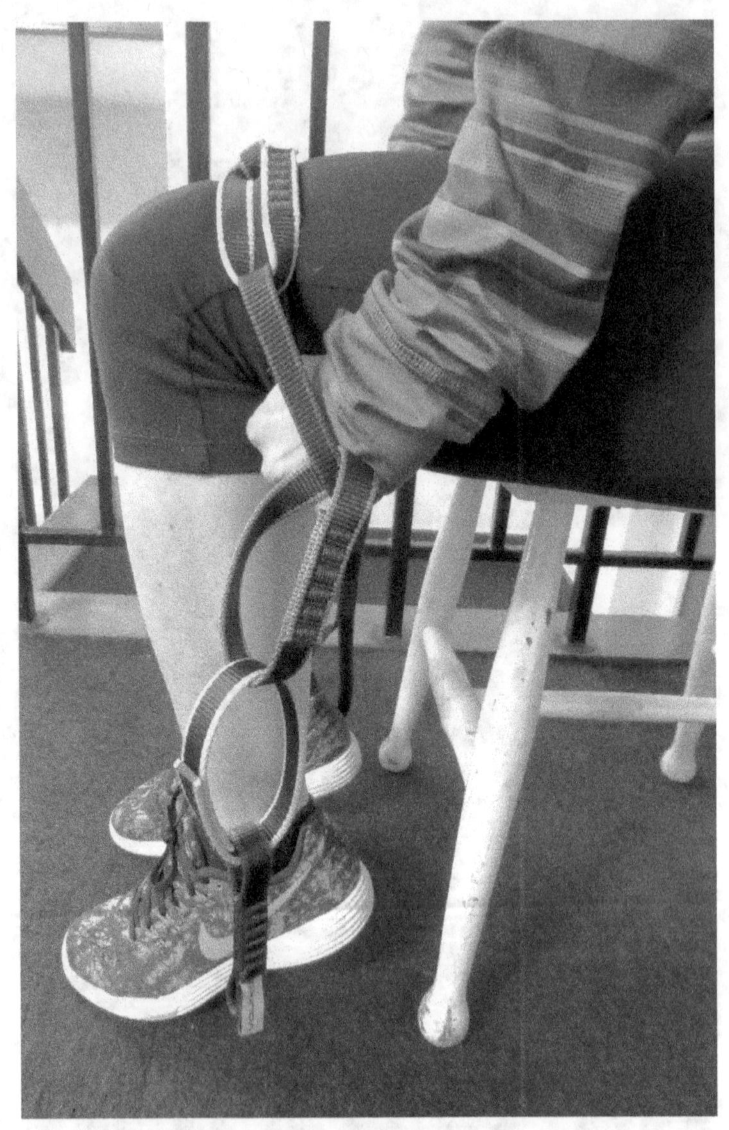

Sections 8 and 9 Thighs Simultaneous Front and Rear: Leg Extension and Leg Curl Combined

This is not necessarily a daisy chain exercise, but it is highly effective, so we have included it. Sit on a bench, stool, or any solid object. Tuck one foot close to the stool and curl your toes back slightly. Tuck your other foot's heel up against the rear foot's toes. In this position, engage the front thighs of the rear foot/leg to press and extend the leg forward. Simultaneously, engage the rear thigh muscles of the forward foot/leg to curl the leg back and resist any movement of the other leg. When you have reached the desired angle and level of applied force, perform the exercise. Advanced variations would be when the exercise is performed at different positions on the ROM, or Range of Motion. When you perform an isometric exercise, never hold your breath. Always breathe deeply and naturally, which will be about 10 full breaths at a rate of about 1 second per breath. Perform each exercise for no less than 7 seconds and no longer than 10. Exercise both legs/sides.

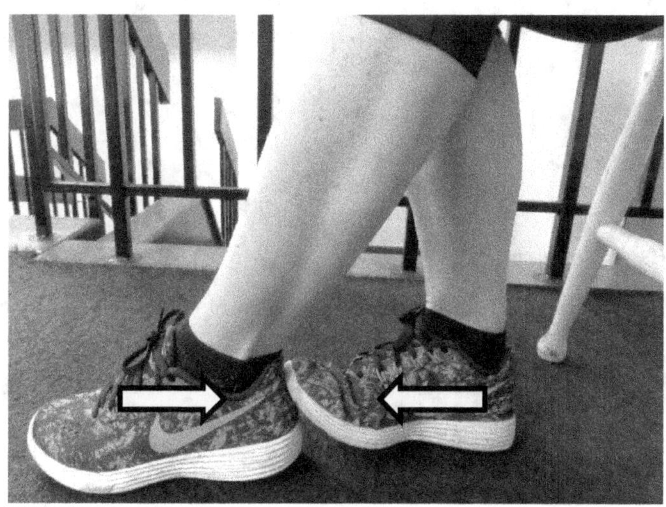

214

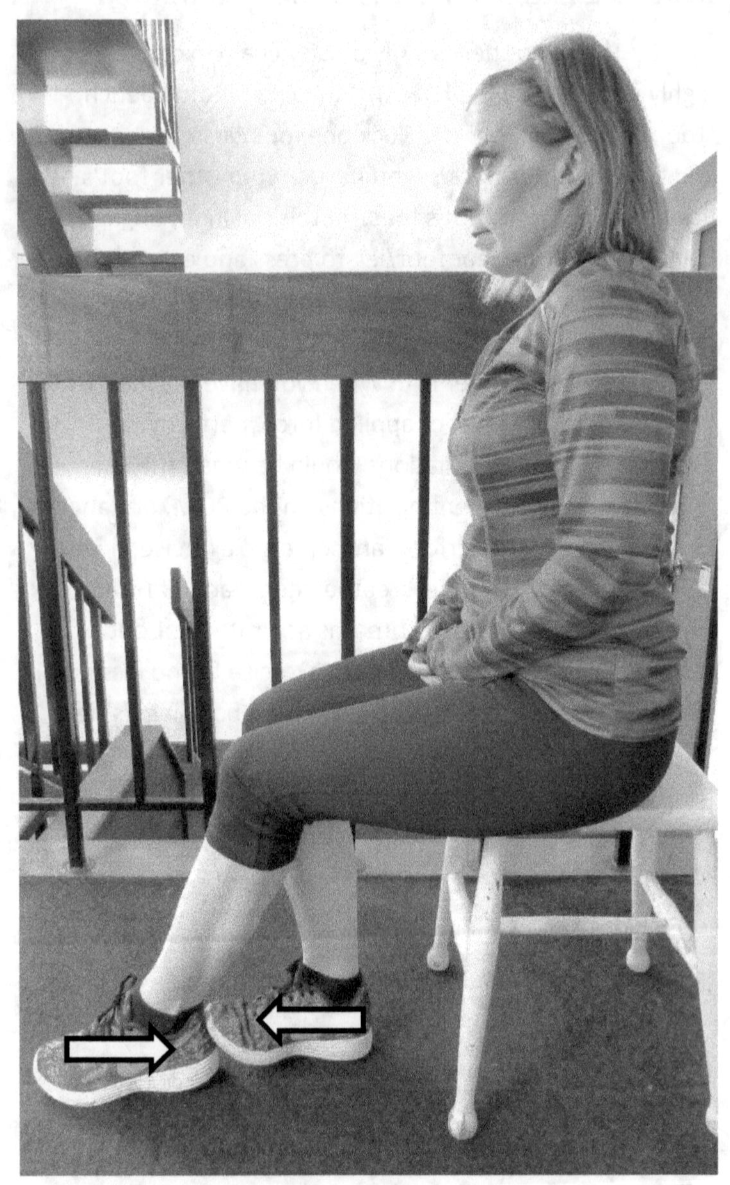

Section 9 Thighs Rear:

Leg Curl Against Wall

This is not necessarily a daisy chain exercise, but it is highly effective, which is why we have included it. Stand with both feet slightly away from a wall or other solid object. In this position, raise one leg slightly to the rear so that the heel meets the wall/object. Always keep your foot and toes pulled up and toward your knee. With your back flat against the wall, attempt to curl your leg by pushing the heel into the wall and upwards to perform the exercise. When you perform an isometric exercise, never hold your breath. Always breathe deeply and naturally, which will be about 10 full breaths at a rate of about 1 second per breath. Perform each exercise for no less than 7 seconds and no longer than 10. Exercise both legs/sides.

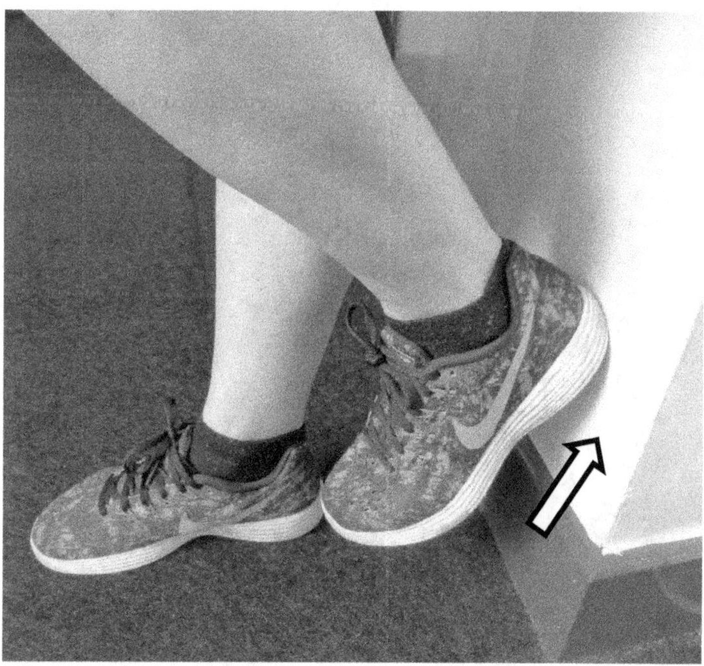

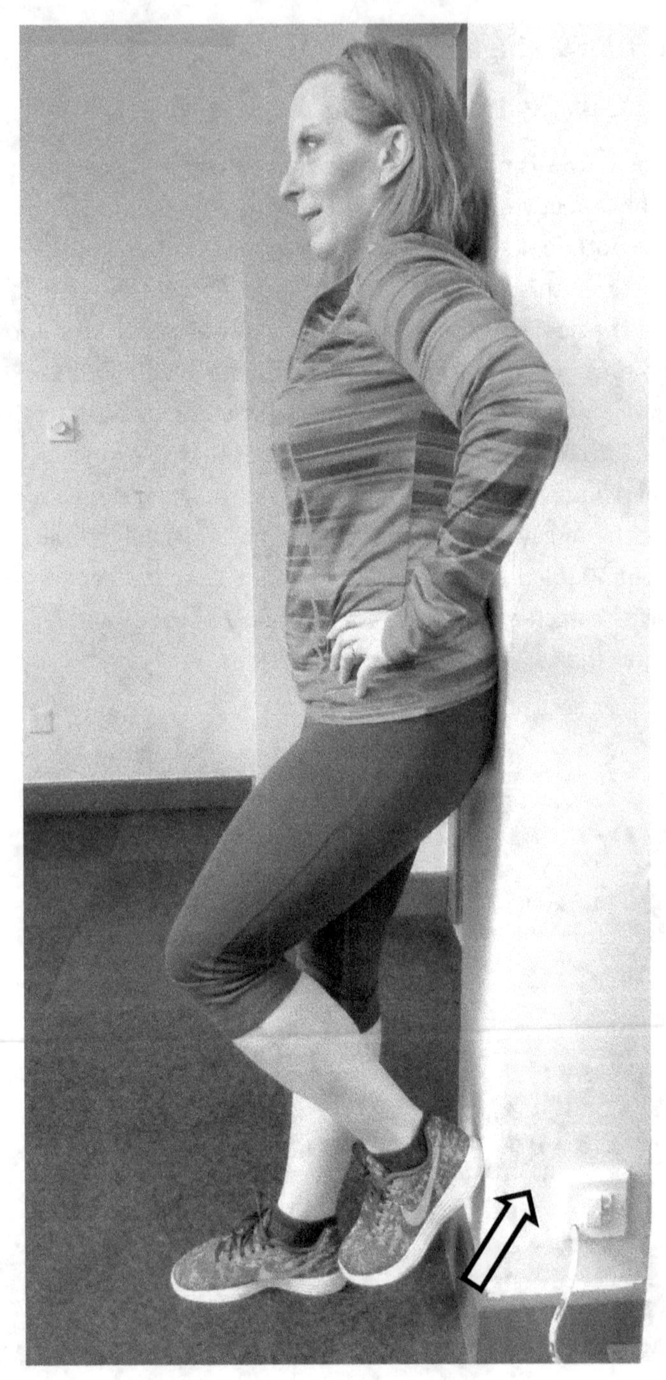

217

Section 10 Calf:

Immovable Object Heel Raise-Push

This is not necessarily a daisy chain exercise, but it is highly effective, which is why we have included it. Stand in front of a wall or any other solid, immovable object at arm's length from you and place the palms of your hands on it. Step backwards with one leg, placing your foot flat on the floor behind you. In this position, use the calf muscles of the rear foot as the driver. Push as you attempt to raise the heel of your foot and move the immovable object to perform the exercise. When you perform an isometric exercise, never hold your breath. Always breathe deeply and naturally, which will be about 10 full breaths at a rate of about 1 second per breath. Perform each exercise for no less than 7 seconds and no longer than 10. Do not forget to exercise both legs.

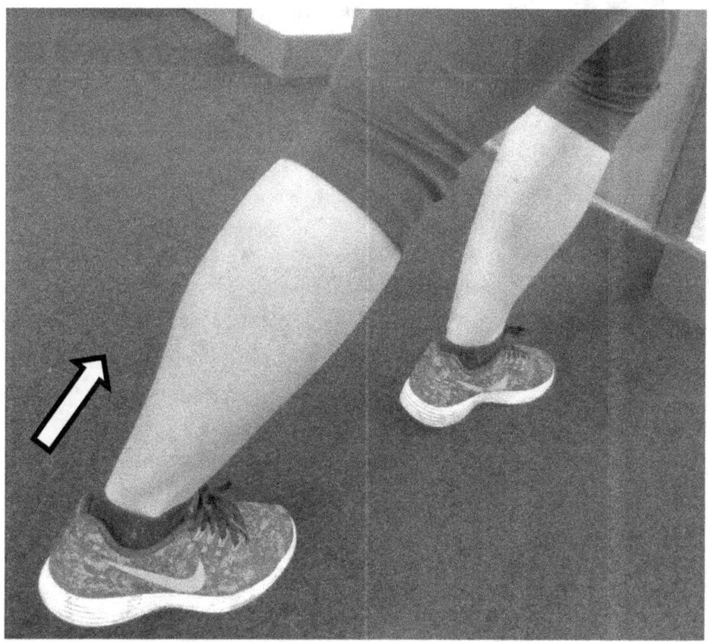

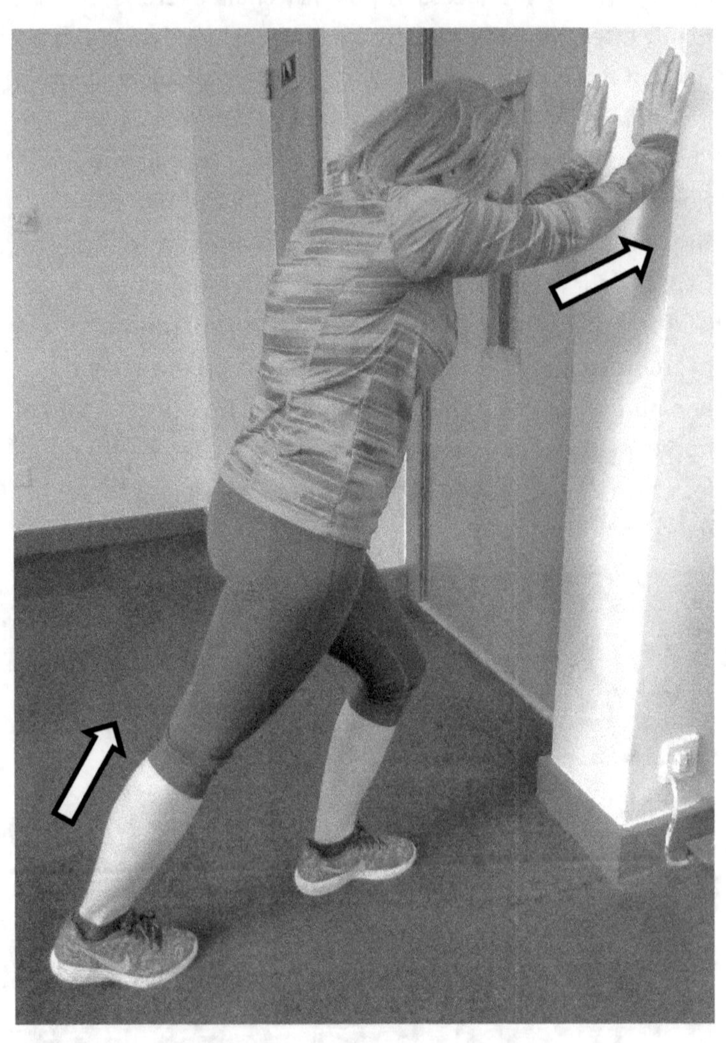

Chapter 7: Conclusion

We sincerely hope that you have found the exercise ideas and variations using daisy chains useful. Daisy chains are an excellent IIED – Improvised Isometric Exercise Device. They are inexpensive, lightweight, strong, portable, versatile, and effective. One of the wonderful things about daisy chains is that they can be easily extended by attaching them to climbing slings and/or other daisy chains either by looping them together or by a carabiner. No matter how strong you are, they are almost impossible to break through human muscle power alone. This means that even the strongest people in the world can use them effectively.

The whole point of an IIED is that it is a common device or object that is structurally robust and easy to use as an effective isometric exercise device, with typically little or no adjustment needed. Daisy chains tick every box in this respect. There are many things in everyday life that can be used effectively as an IIED.

To discover more, you simply need to keep an open and creative mind when going about your daily life. This way, new ideas for IIEDs will be revealed regularly. The better your understanding of biomechanics, the easier it will be to spot many more potential IIEDs. Also, you will be able to perform many more exercises more effectively with any IIED.

Always think about safety first, and never use something that may be structurally unsound, making it likely to break or fail if used as an IIED.

As we find, trial, and approve more IIEDs, we will create new resource books about them. Even though you do not need any special equipment or devices to perform an effective total-body isometric workout, it does not mean that you should not use some if you wish. Using some equipment can be beneficial at times, especially for the more advanced users who want to perform a wider range of exercises at higher levels of intensity.

Also, using IIEDs can make an isometric exercise session much more fun, varied, and interesting. When you find something new that you think has merit and is safe to use, give it a try. If it works, let us know and share the idea with others! We wish you success and good luck in your exercise quest and life in general.

What is TWiEA™?

TWiEA™ is the acronym for The World Isometric Exercise Association. Its mission is to help set and maintain standards of excellence in teaching and promoting all types of isometric exercise. It seeks to ensure that scientifically proven isometric exercise techniques are taught as part of an integrated total-body exercise solution provided by fitness professionals. This increases the probability that busy clients facing real-life time crunches can maintain an effective exercise program. Isometric exercise is every bit as effective at building muscle and strength as other traditional forms of resistance training. It is also a time— and money-saving exercise solution that almost anyone can perform without any special equipment.

Other books by Brian Sterling-Vete and Helen Renée Wuorio

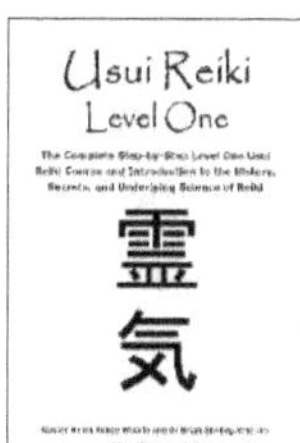

Usui Reiki Level One

An introduction to Reiki, covering its history and supporting science, is presented in an easy step-by-step format. This book and others in the series are course manuals for our online or in-person students.

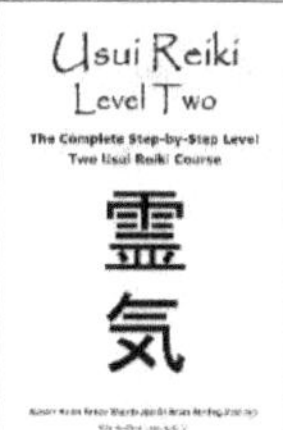

Usui Reiki Level Two

The Reiki Level Two course advances your journey, teaching Power Symbols and their usage. It excludes the history and science from book one and is structured logically in a clear, step-by-step format.

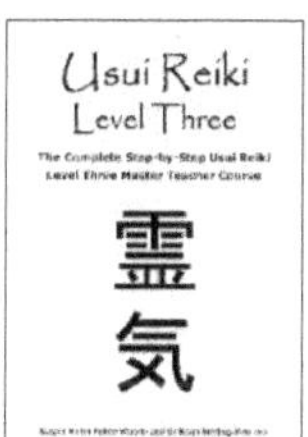

Usui Reiki Level Three

The Level Three Master Teacher course finalises the journey for Level Two practitioners. It focuses solely on Level Three concepts organised in a step-by-step format.

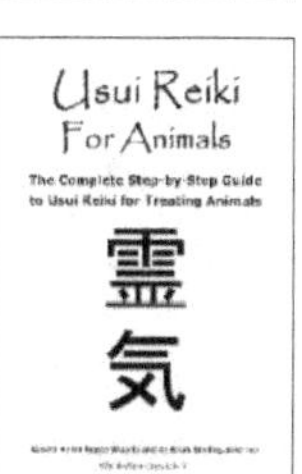

Usui Reiki Compendium (Levels One & Two)

The Reiki Compendium is a complete book of our Level One and Two courses, ideal for anyone wanting to progress through all levels of their Reiki Journey. It also serves as a manual for our students.

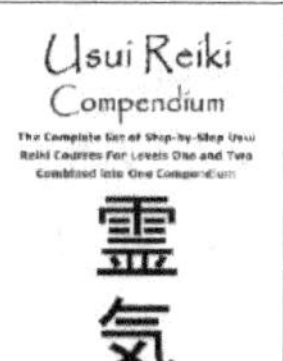

Usui Reiki for Treating Animals

This is perfect for practitioners of all levels wanting to learn safe and effective treatment technique, chakras and energy centres unique to specific animals.

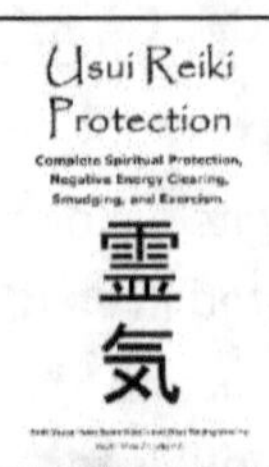

Usui Reiki Protection

The complete guide to spiritual protection, negative energy clearing, smudging, and exorcism, essential for every paranormal investigator and anyone wishing to clear people and places of negative energy.

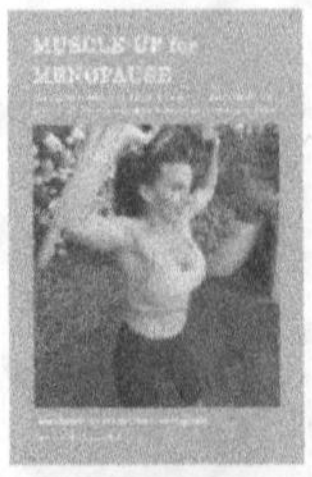

Muscle-up For Menopause

Menopause is inevitable, so take control. Brief, intense exercises with minimal recovery demands and a high-protein plant-based diet positively impact your menopause experience.

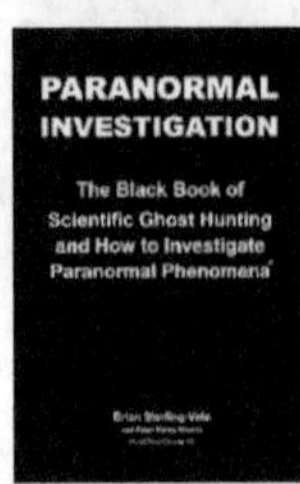

Paranormal Investigation - The Black Book of Scientific Ghost Hunting

It contains a scientific critical path graphic to work from and a step-by-step guide to a complete professional paranormal investigation.

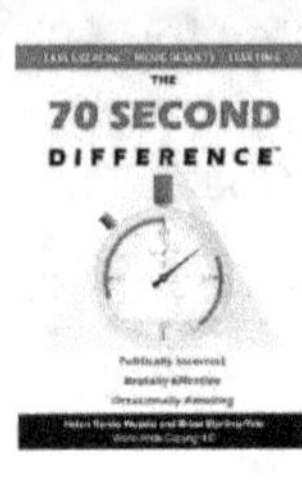

The 70 Second Difference - Politically Incorrect, Occasionally Amusing, and Brutally Effective

Just 70 seconds of focused science-based daily exercise can provide a total-body workout.

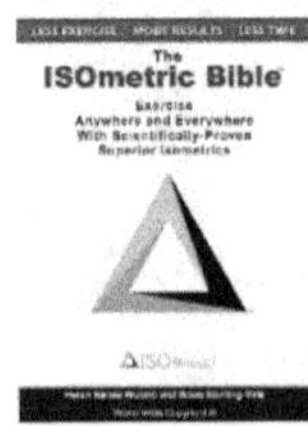

The ISOmetric Bible - Exercise Anywhere with Scientifically Proven Isometrics

A complete, scientific, and user-friendly benchmark book about scientifically proven isometric exercises: no special equipment is needed for a total-body workout.

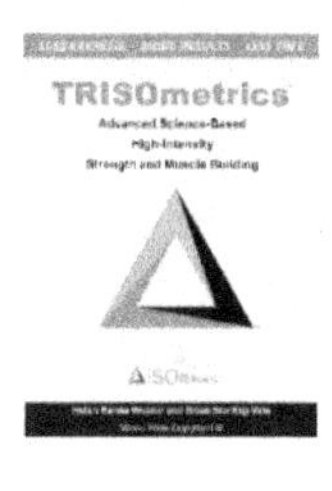

TRISOmetrics - Advanced Science-Based High-Intensity Strength and Muscle Building
This advanced, high-intensity exercise system combines three proven techniques into a powerful new approach, with or without equipment, while travelling or in the gym.

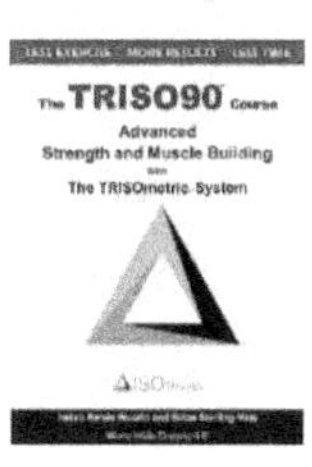

The TRISO90 Course – Advanced Strength and Muscle Building with TRISOmetrics.
A 90-day step-by-step advanced bodybuilding and strength-training course performed with or without equipment or in a gym routine.

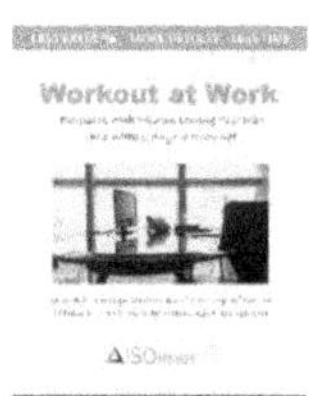

Workout at Work - Exercise at Work Without Anyone Even Knowing What You're Doing!
Science-based Isometric exercises let you work out effectively and discreetly without leaving your desk.

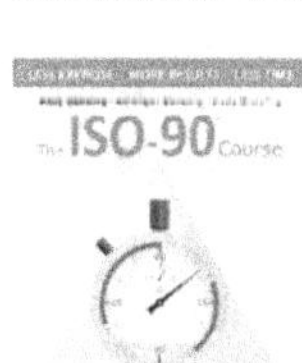

The ISO90 Course – The 12-Week/90-Day Shape-up and Get Strong Course. A complete step-by-step 90-day isometric body shaping, bodybuilding, and strength-building course is ideal for both beginners and advanced.

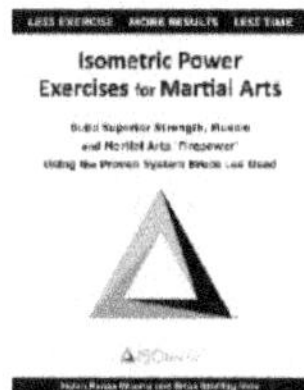

Isometric Power Exercises for Martial Arts - Build Superior Strength, Muscle and Martial Arts 'Firepower' Using the Proven System Bruce Lee Used. This is a valuable resource for practical isometric exercises that build serious strength, muscle, and martial arts firepower.

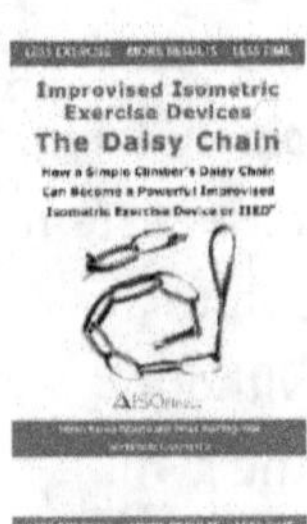

Improvised Isometric Exercise Devices (IIEDs) - The Daisy Chain

This is a resource for practical exercises that can be performed and for learning how to extend the daisy chain safely.

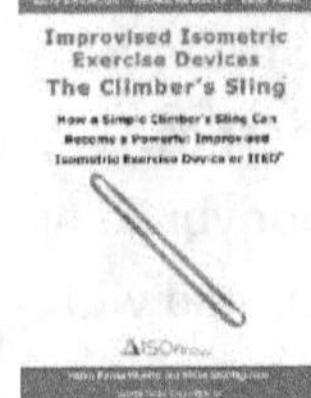

Improvised Isometric Exercise Devices (IIEDs) - The Climber's Sling

This valuable resource lists practical isometric exercises that can be performed and how to safely extend the climber's sling.

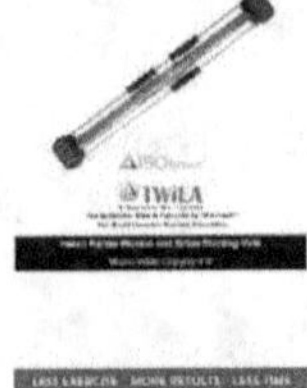

The Bullworker Bible - The Ultimate Science-Based Guide to The Classic Personal Multi-Gym. Approved by Bullworker.com. It is a complete, science-based user-friendly book and companion to The Bullworker 90 Course.

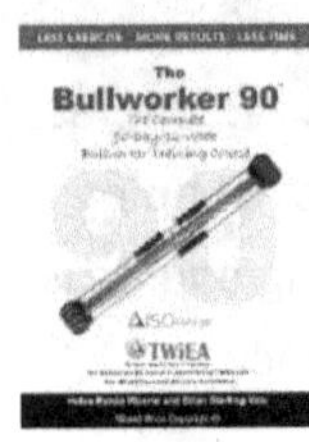

The Bullworker 90™ Course - The Ultimate Science-Based 12-Week/90-Day Get Strong and Grow Muscle Course Approved by The Bullworker makers, this complete 90-day course and companion book to The Bullworker Bible.

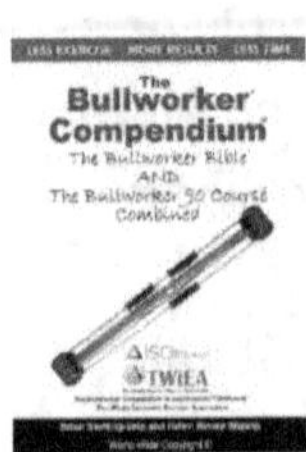

The Bullworker Compendium - The Bullworker Bible and The Bullworker90 Course Combined

Approved by the makers of The Bullworker. The Bullworker Compendium™ combines both The Bullworker Bible™ and The Bullworker 90™ Course in a single huge book.

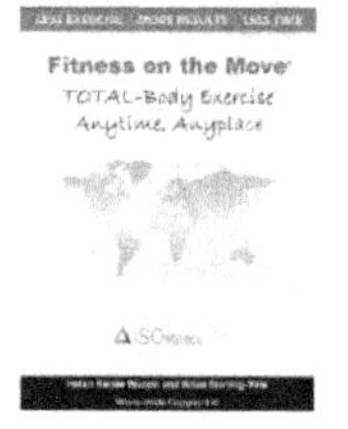

Fitness on the Move

Practical exercises that can be performed while travelling almost anywhere, even in a vehicle. If there is enough space to sit and stand, you can have a total-body workout!

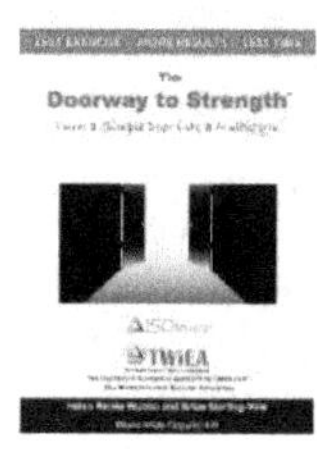

The Doorway to Strength - Turn a Door into a Strength-Building Multigym. It shows how a simple door, doorway, and frame can create a multi-gym of exercises using the amazing Iso-Bow®. Required: 2 x Iso-Bows®, a solid door and frame, and a door wedge/stop.

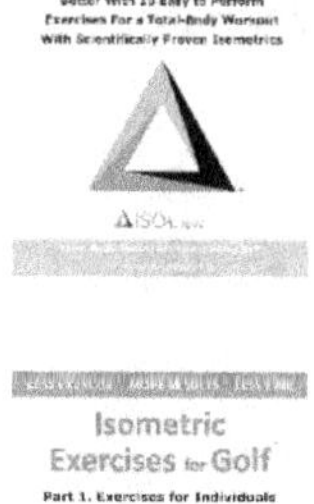

Feel Better In 70 Seconds

Studies show that brief exercise combats depression without significant cost or time. Just 70 seconds of continuous movement allows a full-body workout using isometric exercises, requiring 2 x Iso-Bows®.

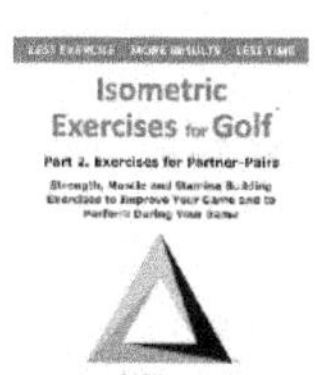

Isometric Exercises for Golf Part 1. Exercises for Individuals. Isometric exercises can turn a round of golf into a full-body workout at each hole, using a golf club as a makeshift exercise tool. Part 1 provides customised exercises to improve swing power for individual needs.

Isometric Exercises for Golf Part 2. Partner-Pairs. The companion to Book 1 focuses on exercises best performed in partnered pairs during breaks, games, or practice sessions.

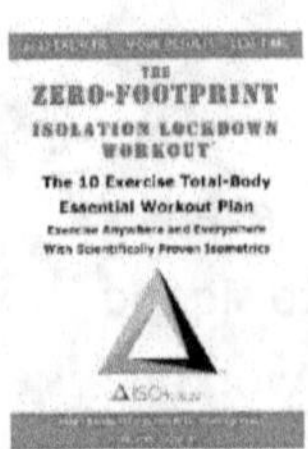
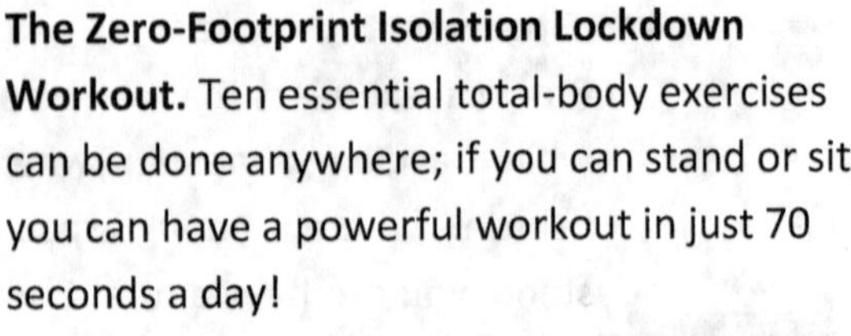

The Zero-Footprint Isolation Lockdown Workout. Ten essential total-body exercises can be done anywhere; if you can stand or sit, you can have a powerful workout in just 70 seconds a day!

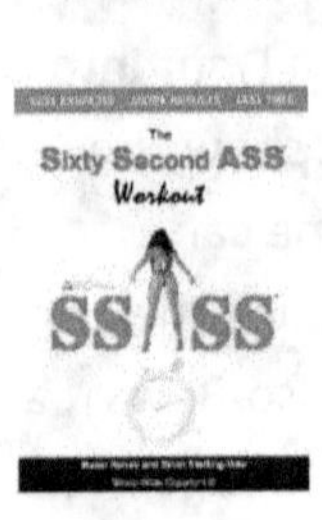

The Sixty Second ASS Workout - Shape, Tone, Lift, and Get the Backside You've Always Wanted. The fastest and most effective "ass" workout ever devised. Scientifically proven exercises deliver a no-nonsense, time-efficient workout.

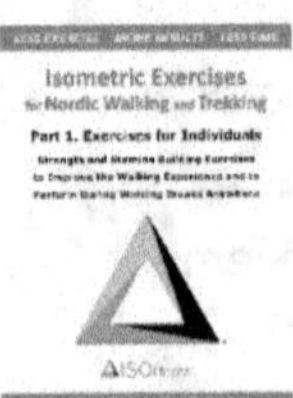

Isometric Exercises for Nordic Walking and Trekking - Part 1. Exercises for Individuals. Perform total-body isometric exercises during walk breaks using walking poles as an Improvised Isometric Exercise Device. Book 1 serves as a resource guide for individuals.

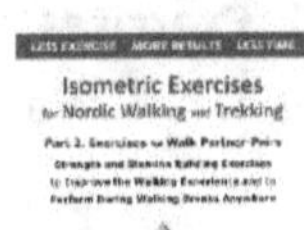
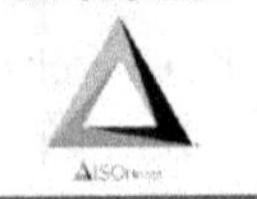

Isometric Exercises for Nordic Walking and Trekking - Part 2. Exercises for Walk Partner-Pairs.
This is the companion to Book 1 focusing on exercises performed as a walking partner.

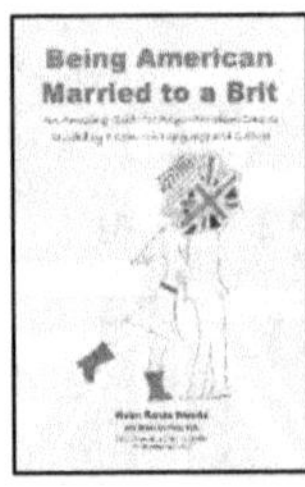

Being American Married to a Brit - An Amusing Guide for Anglo-American Couples. This quirky, fun-filled roller coaster ride is about how even the most basic everyday transatlantic conversations can bring laughter. It's dedicated to all transatlantic couples.

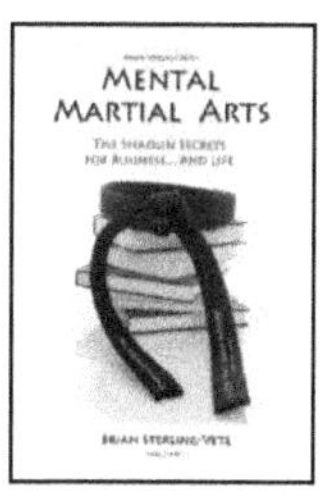

Mental Martial Arts - Intellectual Life and Business Combat Skills. An intellectual language and combat skills system based on martial arts principles. Learn to guide and redirect the energy of influential individuals and large organisations to achieve goals.

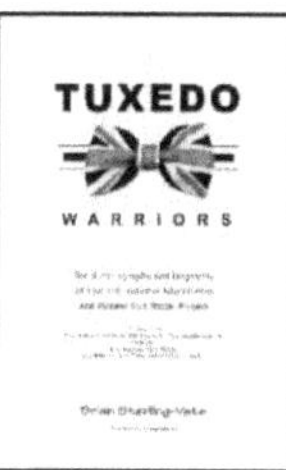

Tuxedo Warriors

The companion book to The Tuxedo Warrior expands on the story, serving as both a biography and autobiography of cult author Cliff Twemlow. It also includes unique insights from Brian Sterling-Vete.

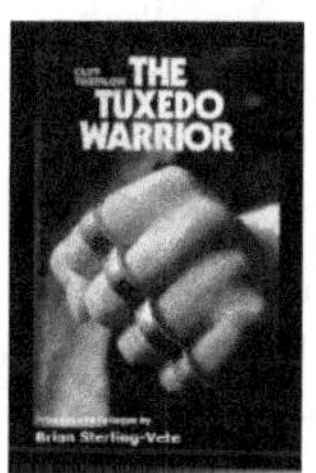

The Tuxedo Warrior by Cliff Twemlow – A doorman manages respect using either diplomacy or force. This requires balancing peaceful solutions with violent encounters, providing a raw perspective on the lively yet perilous world of clubland peacekeeping.

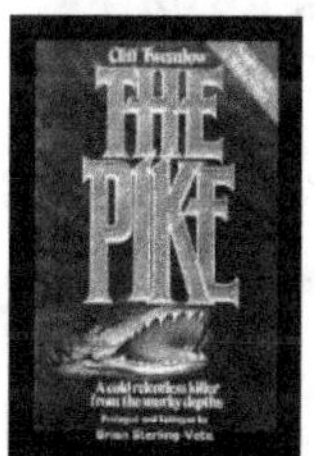

The Pike by Cliff Twemlow – A monstrous pike terrorises Lake Windermere, attacking people and boats, causing panic. Some exploit the chaos, hindering the creature's capture to profit as the terror escalates.

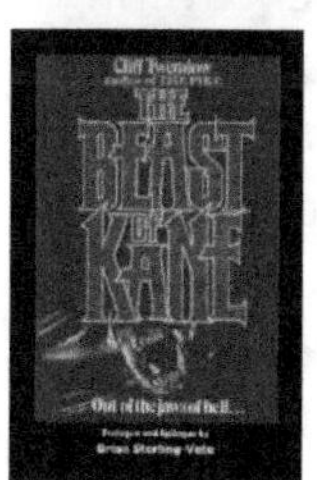

The Beast of Kane by Cliff Twemlow – The Gordon family invites darkness by adopting a stray Elkhound, igniting ancient evil prophecies. Kane faces supernatural terror, from animal attacks to gruesome murder, as a chilling winter amplifies the fear in town.

228

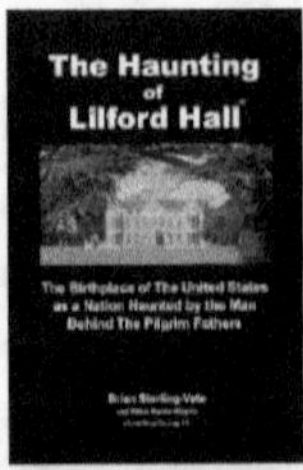

The Haunting of Lilford Hall - The Birthplace of the United States as a Nation Haunted by the Man Behind The Pilgrim Fathers. A baffling case of paranormal activity occurred from 2012 to 2013, involving multiple people.

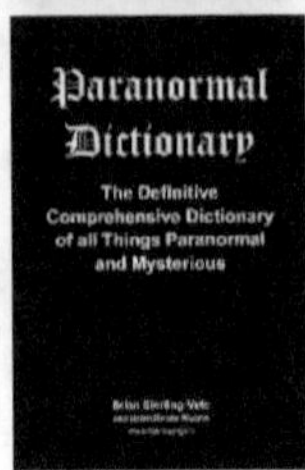

Paranormal Dictionary

This comprehensive guide covers the most common paranormal terminology, entities, and equipment used during investigations. Ideal for both new and experienced investigators.

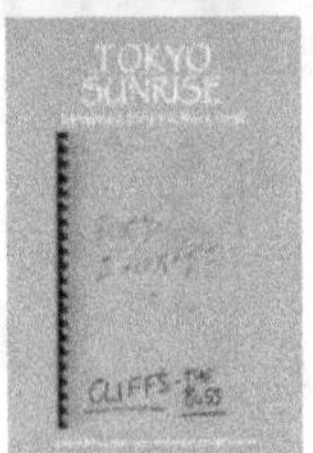

Tokyo Sunrise Background Story and Script

One of Cliff Twemlow's famous film concepts. Cinematographer Robert Foster produced a promotional sizzle reel, aiming to sell the movie to potential investors. This also tells the story of the Richard Gere connection.

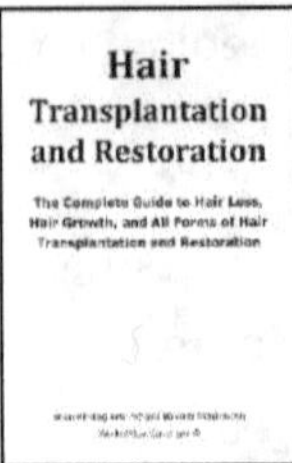

Hair Transplantation and Restoration

The essential guide to hair loss, growth, and ALL forms of hair transplantation and restoration. Malcolm Mendelsohn is the world's #1 independent expert with almost 50 years of experience.

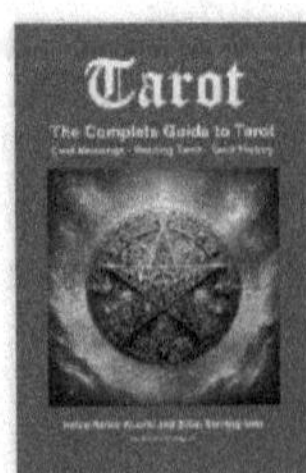

Tarot – The Complete Guide

Explore the ultimate tarot guide, covering its history, card styles, and meanings. Master the art and science of tarot reading with insights and secret techniques from an internationally acclaimed Tarot Master, Helen Renée.

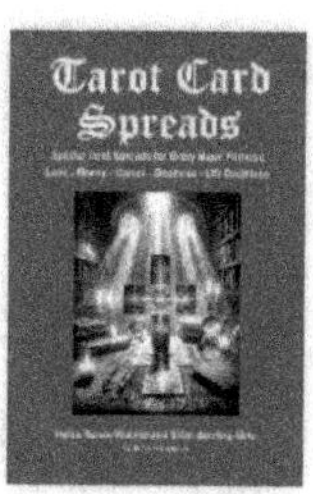

Tarot Card Spreads

Discover the ultimate tarot spread guide, featuring various spreads for love, money, career, business, and key life decisions. It includes detailed diagrams and descriptions to enhance your tarot practice.

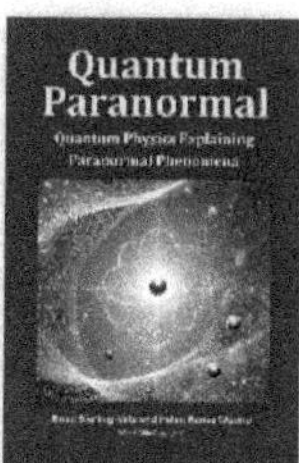

Quantum Paranormal

Quantum physics meets the paranormal, offering fascinating explanations about the existence of paranormal phenomena and the mechanisms underpinning them. This deeply controversial book also challenges a crucial belief at the foundation of the Christian Church.